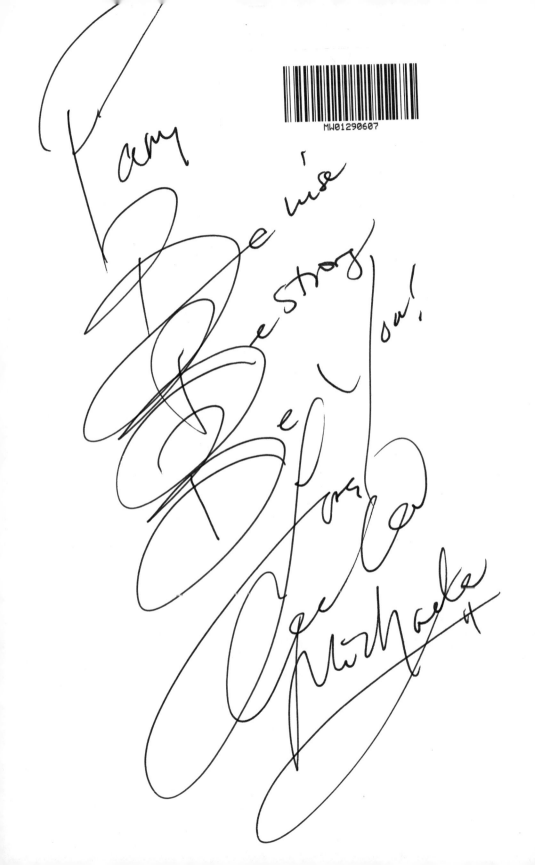

Larry
Be wise
Be strong
Be you!
Love
Gee Michaele

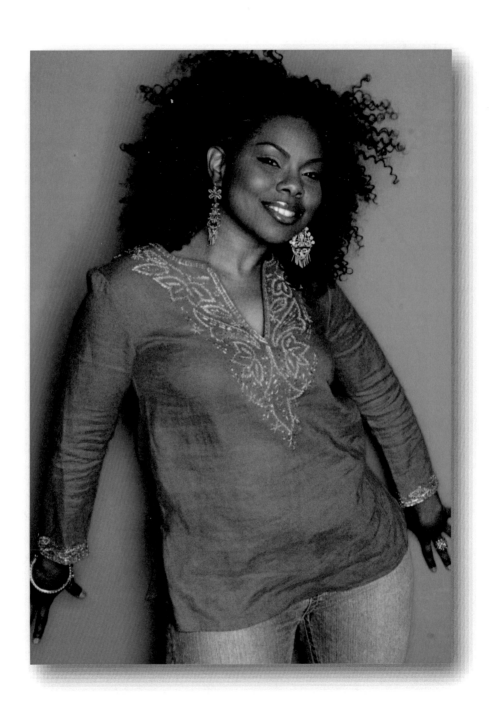

ZULEANA ®

NEW WAY OF LIFE

Cee Cee Michaela

ZULEANA®A New Way of Life
Copyright © 2017 by Cee Cee Michaela
ISBN-13:978-1548696276
ISBN-10:1548696277
Nutrition/Health/Wellness
First printing 2017
Printed and bound in the United States of America.

Zuleana® is a registered trademark of Michaela's Creativity Studio,
LLC, a Cee Cee Michaela company.
Cover photo: Derek Blanks
Wedding photo: Rachel Fesko
All other photos: Cee Cee Michaela and Wilbert Floyd
(except before and after photos)

Quantity discounts are available on bulk purchases of this book for
educational, gift purchases or as premiums. For information please e-mail:
ceecee@zuleana.com

The information in this book is not intended nor implied to be a substitute for
professional medical advice, diagnosis or treatments. All content, including
text, graphics, images and information contained on or available through this
book, is for general information only. The author makes no representation and
assumes no responsibility for the accuracy of information contained in this
book. Nor for any loss or damage of any nature suffered as a result of reliance
on any of this book's contents or errors or omissions herein. You are
encouraged to review all information regarding any medical condition or
treatment with your physician.

*T*his book is dedicated to my mom, Vivian Patterson, a vibrant, 81-year-old character. Who wants to write another *"In Loving Memory of"* book? Not me! I want to honor my mother while she still lives— and that

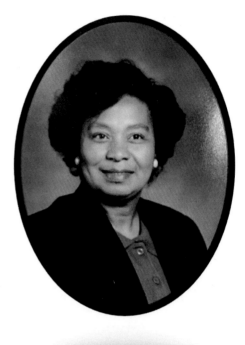

she does. She was an English teacher for 30 years and still teaches reading skills to preschoolers to this day. She is a hoot and always keeps my sisters and me in stiches as she tells familial memories, using elaborate facial expressions and exquisitely colorful, storytelling vocal tones. My amazing, octogenarian mom is strong and wise. In my opinion, she is the best mom ever. This book is also dedicated to all those who have an ear to hear. Those who choose life and not death. Those who want to ***eat to live and not live to eat!***

Acknowledgements

*T*o my *Lord* and *Savior*, for choosing me and giving me constant assignments. Thank You, Lord, for everything. I am so in love with You!

To my sweet and witty nephew, JaGerran Knight, you inspire me. Your smile and drive motivate me to make sure you and millions of others like you, know more about the power of natural health.

To Dackeyia Sterling for watching my Facebook posts, then hitting me up on my Facebook and saying, "You wanna write a book? Call me!" This is now the third book that I have written in three years after that life-changing phone call. Wow!

To my sister friend, Janet N. Love. I can hear you now saying, "Shut the front door!" And to my friend girl, Cassandra Haire. I know this book will make you feel your "SHA NA NA NA!" A special thank you to Rashatta Daugett who is always there for me through every circumstance. You are so dear to me and I am thankful to call you friend. May God continue to bless your socks off!

To all the Zuleana® Girls across the US who have joined me on this Zuleana® underground journey. Thank you for being so dedicated to the movement. Your diligence is deeply appreciated and the results show all over you! You ladies are so beautiful and practically *"zuleana skinny"* now!   #zuleanamakesyoudisappear

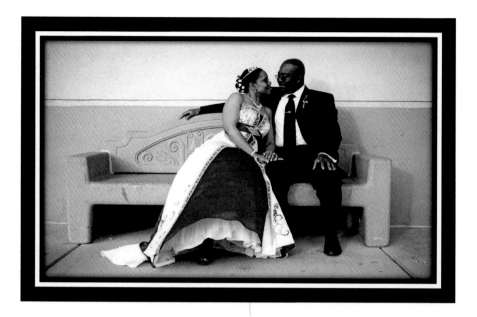

L ast, but not least, I thank my husband, Wilbert. Your loving kindness, patience, and wisdom blow me away. I celebrate, honor, and appreciate you, Papa Bear! I am so excited to be your MRS. and I'm very grateful that you are diggin' this whole natural health lifestyle. You took to it pretty quickly and now you are practically a *Zuleana® beast*!

Thanks for working so hard. You would practically find a thousand ways to make my never-ending bucket list come true. I love seeing you snag product from the shipment and willingly test out my healthy goodness. From Chinese guava leaf tea to delicious mangosteen tea from Thailand, you wake up and go to bed totally dedicated to consuming your healthy elixirs and this makes me super happy. I can only hope to be like you when I grow up. LOL. But no... like, for real though! Year after year, our love just keeps on growing. You are truly my *endless love.*

Zuleana® (zu leen´ ah) noun: a healthy living

lifestyle concept, created by

Cee Cee Michaela.

The *Zu* was inspired by the Zulu tribe out of

Africa. It's the way in which we dance and

move.

The *Lean* is how the body looks when one

follows the Zuleana® way of healthy eating.

The results make the body more LEAN,

especially in the waistline.

It's a way of eating, a style of dancing,

a sisterhood, a movement.

This is... 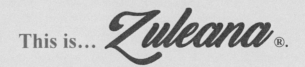®.

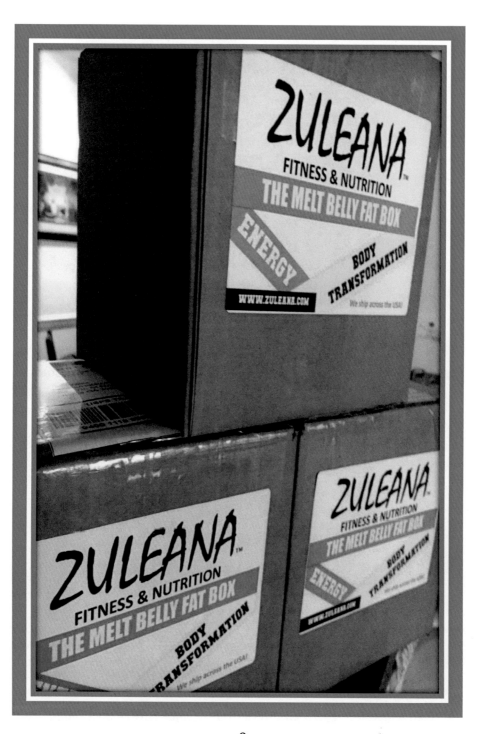

A Note from the Author

The Melt Belly Fat Box
A 3-Piece Weight Loss System

S o many of you may have either seen my Zuleana® Facebook Live videos, my Zuleana® Life TV YouTube videos, or heard me speak at a women's conference. Some of you may have already experienced a brand new lifestyle by tapping into the amazing Zuleana® system. Maybe you have never met me before but you have already visited my website: **www.Zuleana.com** and ordered your personal one-on-one Zuleana® better health consultation. Maybe we have had the chance to laugh, cry, and cackle over the phone as we came up with a customized eating and supplements plan that finally laid your health concerns to rest!

It has truly been an honor to serve you for all of these years. I am slowly rising to be known as the "go-to girl" for all things pure and natural of the World Wide Web. I am blown away by the customers' excitement when they visit my online store and are able to find everything from chemical-free nail polish in a beautiful exotic floral color to crazy-affordable, 99% cacao dark chocolate. I am talking one dollar, folks!

Out of all of my years of *medicine hunting*, the green anti-eczema soap is a top seller. It gets rid of eczema so quickly and effectively that I will probably never ever discontinue this coveted blessing that kills tormenting scratch-and-itch demons of the underworld upon contact. But

I must admit, we have a problem, America. Whether you call it a muffin top, love handles or the tire, it seems like everyone wants to lose belly fat.

Over all of my years of collecting the best of the best in all-natural health products, packing your items with lots of tender care and lots of prayer, and shipping them quickly to your front door, I have never seen an item sell as well as my famous **Melt Belly Fat Box**. It is an easy 3-piece weight loss system that includes the following:

1. Japanese matcha green tea powder, which you drink first thing in the morning

2. Artichoke leaf tea, which you drink in the afternoon

3. White by night gentle detox powder, which you mix with water and drink right before you go to bed

These three powerful, all-natural items help to burn the belly fat, clean the amyloid plaque from the brain, increase energy and stamina, cleanse the skin, liver, and gallbladder, and lower bad cholesterol. It also flushes out old fecal matter, parasites, yeast/candida, bacteria, and heavy metals from the body. The Melt Belly Fat Box definitely works and you will get to see Zuleana® weight loss before and after pictures and testimonies a little later in this book.

Now, when was the last time you really took time out for yourself to do what we call in Zuleana®, *self-care?* There is only one you! Your body has been given to you to run, jump, play, move, bend, and sway, as you please. You were created to lift your hands, not only to pray, but to sew and to cook, to carve and to paint. Imagine working with your hands,

Using kaleidoscope-colored sea glass from California, West African elephant grass, or Thai purple silk, and allowing these elements to slip through your busy, creative fingers with ease. What about hiking the mountains of Colorado or swimming with the dolphins in Aruba?

Yes! Zuleana® girls are dropping pounds and dropping meds all across the U.S. and we are having fun. Their Zuleana® husbands are obtaining better health results by default through their wives' better health choices and all the little Zuleana® children are living happily ever after. Zuleana® is a sisterhood. It is a beautiful community that is growing like wildfire and whenever we all meet up, we are simply unstoppable!

I am Cee Cee Michaela, the creator of Zuleana®. I am excited to share my knowledge and worth with you. We can and we will be free from sickness and disease together, because I know the way. I am your natural health conductor and we are gonna ride this natural health train until the wheels fall all the way off. And even then, we will transform the wheels into floating devices and start *rolling on the river.*
Welcome to ZULEANA® ...a new way of life!

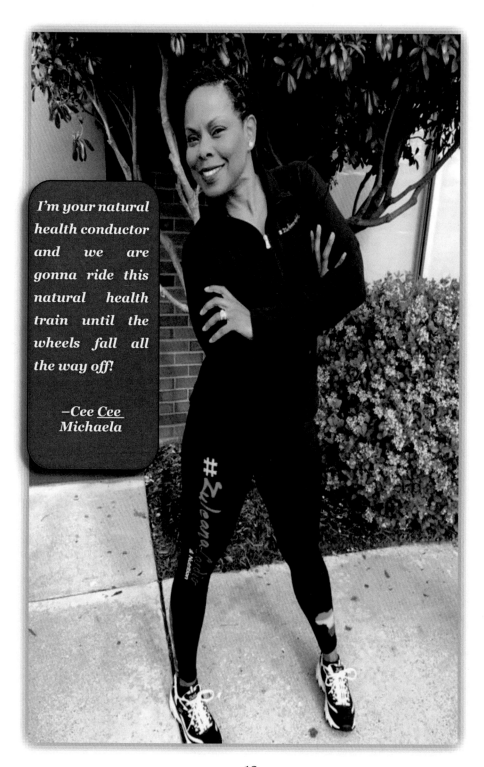

I'm your natural health conductor and we are gonna ride this natural health train until the wheels fall all the way off!

—Cee Cee Michaela

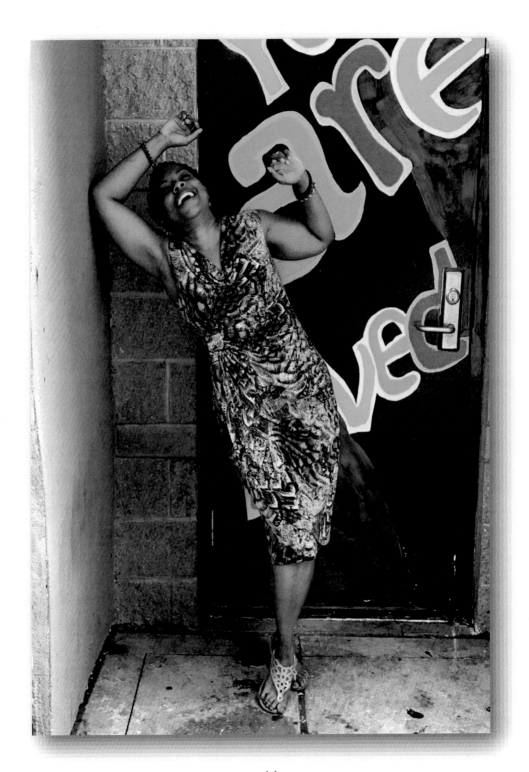

14

Zuleana® Poem #1: You Are

You are brilliant
You are resilient
You are resourceful
You are unencumbered
You are someone's sunshine
You are the reason trees breathe
You are the master's handiwork
You are a cup that runs over
You are clay in the potter's hand
You are a runner in this race
You are a good thing
You are healed
You are free

You Are Loved

**Poem inspired by a beautiful door on Hargett Street in Raleigh, NC.

Introduction

How Zuleana® Began

I was about 23 years old when I was casted in a production and relocated to Toronto, Ontario Canada, at the fabulous St. Lawrence Center for the Arts. I played a sweet, bright-eyed, dark-skinned ingenue by the name of Ti Moune in a Caribbean-infused musical entitled "Once on This Island." Downtown Toronto was so much fun and was incredibly clean compared to what I was use to while living in Manhattan. One of my fellow cast members, who happened to be my age, was a vegan. I didn't want to hang with the older crowd nor eat solo, so I decided to eat the way that she ate, whatever this "vegan stuff" was, in order to not offend her. A bit skeptical, I took a bite of something I thought was meat and it turned out to be vegetables. It was absolutely delicious and I have been hooked on healthy eating ever since. My contract with this show lasted for about six months, then it was time to return to the U.S. Needless to say, I had a little more money in my pocket and a lot less toxins and junk food in my digestive system. I could not go back to my old way of eating.

Well, here I am, 23 years later, and I have created my very own clean eating lifestyle called Zuleana®. It's a far cry from the hard-core vegan eating of my younger days. That was much too limited for me. I began to study herbs, leaves, barks, spices, supplements, vitamins, and minerals. After many years of rigorous and tireless research, collecting some of the best natural medicines and helping thousands in the U.S.to heal their ailments naturally, I began to accept invitations from across the world to speak and teach natural health workshops! Yes, I have had the opportunity to perform a Japanese tea ceremony to the native, sweet-hearted, centurion women in Sasebo, Japan. I have also taught a three-hour natural health interactive seminar to beautiful, inquisitive, Caribbean girls set along the white sands of the beach on the beautiful island of St. Lucia. I absolutely love what I do.

My name is Cee Cee Michaela, but I am affectionately known as the *"Harriet Tubman of Health"* and I know without a doubt that my calling and personal mission is to make sure that I gently push people out of the bondage of sickness and disease and carry them to freedom through the awareness of foods that harm and foods that heal. I know that so many of you want to lose weight but you don't know exactly what to eat. You want your disease to go away using natural elements, but you don't know what to consume to really eradicate the disease forever. I knew my anti-fat, anti-disease lifestyle must be highly effective, extremely doable, and well…downright tasty. Zuleana® is a new way of eating that you will love for a lifetime. Zuleana® meals include clean water, healthy oils, a few meats, lots of spices, plenty of fruit, vegetables, and yes, even dark chocolate…yuuumm! So let the *Zuleana® way* begin.

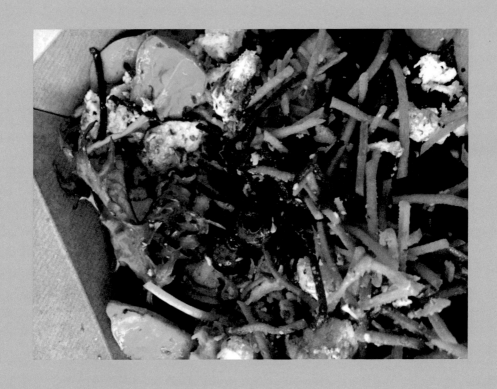

Zuleana® is a new way of eating that you will love for a lifetime.

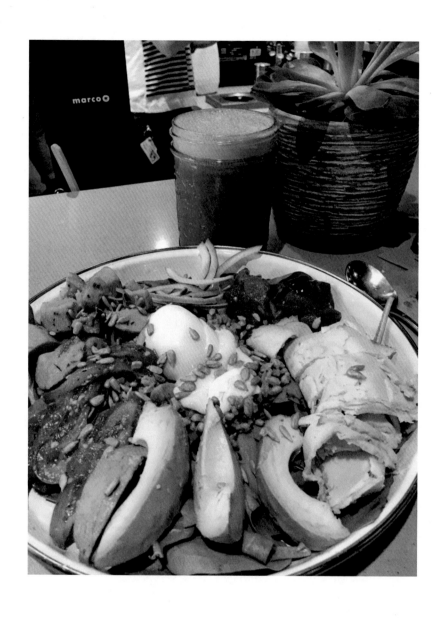

I knew my anti-fat, anti-disease lifestyle must be highly effective, extremely doable and well...
downright tasty.

What Makes Zuleana® So Special

What if you knew that every food that you eat actually releases nutrition and that same nutrition could heal you naturally? What if you knew that eating a red apple would bring you less stress while a green apple is lower in calories? The skin of red grapes is healthier than the skin of green grapes! Broccoli helps fight cancer! There is yellow spice from India that you can eat and drink every day that helps take away massive inflammation and pain out of your joints, stops cancer from moving and keeps your brain healthy and sharp with tons of nothing but fabulous gray matter!

This is what makes Zuleana® so different. You are not only going to learn **what** to eat but **when** to eat it and **why** you are eating it. Did you know that it's best to eat blueberries in the morning and cherries and kiwi at night? Or, how about if you sleep with all of the lights off, you will produce a hormone that will help you sleep better, lose weight and possibly help fight cancer? Who knew? You do, now! And there is so much more to learn because Zuleana® is so amazingly nutrient-dense and easy to apply to your life. You will discover that you are not only what you eat, but what you drink and consume! What time of the day or evening that you eat certain foods and the portion size of your foods are going to make all the Zuleana® difference!

Zuleana® causes you to become acutely aware of your body and how it works and you will act quickly when something feels a bit off or unusual. Like Hippocrates said, "Let thy food be thy medicine and medicine be thy food." You will finally for once in your life be what we Zuleana® girls like to call a *"mindful" eater*! My new anti-fat, anti-disease lifestyle will give you a sharpened mind, rejuvenated spirit and a bangin' body! It all starts with... shhhhh, come closer. It's a secret…the ***hidden figures.***

The Hidden Figures

Our favorite numbers in Zuleana® are 3, 30, and 60. In the Zuleana® way, we eat three healthy meals and three healthy snacks. We start out with a breakfast, consisting of a bowl of fresh, gluten-free, steel-cut oatmeal topped with ½ cup of blueberries, blackberries, or raspberries. Blueberries have one of the highest levels of polyphenols, which release energy to your cells, so berries are awesome for that amazing pick-me-up in the morning. Place a few ounces of 30-calorie almond milk and ½ teaspoon of Ceylon cinnamon in your oatmeal. Drink another 6-8 ounces of almond milk with ½ teaspoon of Ceylon cinnamon to get your intake of calcium. We call this cinnamon milk. Oooh! Yeah! A super cool idea!

For lunch you will eat one large dark, green leafy salad with lots of antioxidant vegetables such as spinach, kale, beets, carrots, broccoli, berries, and/or romaine lettuce. Top it with 4 ounces of organic chicken, turkey, wild caught salmon or wild caught albacore tuna. Be sure to use a vinaigrette dressing that is no more than 30-60 calories.

We actually make our own Zuleana® dressing but we will get to that recipe a little later. Your three healthy snacks are the following: two apples or an apple and a pear and a 100 calorie snack bag of (17-20) raw almonds, which may be eaten throughout the day.

For dinner you should have 4 oz. of organic chicken, turkey, or wild caught salmon along with brown rice, quinoa or cauliflower rice. Half of your plate should be filled with vegetables such as: sautéed spinach, asparagus, collard greens, turnip greens, cabbage, brussels sprouts, broccoli, cauliflower, yellow squash, zucchini, carrots, butternut squash, or a small sweet potato. Just make sure your meat portions are always 4 oz. Four ounces is the size of a deck of cards or your fist.

In the Zuleana® way, we eat 1,200 calories a day and we do our best to burn a minimum of 500 calories or more with vigorous exercise every day. And one last shocker; try your best not to eat any beans. I know! I was taken aback when I learned this, too! You see that's the problem with…shhhh, come closer. It's a secret…***coming to America!***

THE ZULEANA® MEAL PLAN

Copyright © 2017 by Cee Cee Michaela
www.Zuleana.com

BREAKFAST	LUNCH	SNACKS	DINNER
¼ cup of steel-cut oatmeal ½ cup of blueberries, blackberries, or raspberries 30 calorie almond milk ½ teaspoon of Ceylon cinnamon Drink another 6 ounces of almond milk with ½ teaspoon of Ceylon cinnamon to get your intake of calcium Other Options are: Egg white veggie omelette in coconut oil Grapefruit with one organic boiled egg NO YOGURT! DO NOT HAVE FRIED EGGS! NO BOXED CEREALS!	One big green leafy salad with Romaine lettuce Kale Spinach Carrots Beets Berries Cucumbers Apricots Vinaigrette dressing Extra virgin olive oil Top with 4 oz. of Skinless chicken Skinless turkey Albacore tuna or ½ Avocado Other options are: Veggie plate with NO BEANS!	One green apple One red apple 100 calories pack or 17-20 raw almonds Other options are 1/2 cup of red grapes ½ grapefruit 3 avocado slices 13 cherries Small kiwi Apricot Carrots Cucumber NO PEANUTS! NO BUTTERS! NO CHEESE! NO CORN! NO POPCORN! NO VEGGIE CHIPS!	4 oz. of: Skinless chicken Skinless turkey Wild caught salmon Albacore tuna 1/2 cup of brown rice or quinoa or cauliflower rice ½ of your whole plate should be veggies! (EAT GREEN!) Broccoli Spinach Cabbage Asparagus Squash/Zucchini Collard greens Turnip Greens 2 TBS. of organic Sauerkraut from a jar NO PASTA! NO SOY! NO VEGGIE BURGERS OUT OF A BOX!

*The words in red indicate a perfect Zuleana™ eating day!

THE ZULEANA® GROCERY LIST

Copyright © 2017 by Cee Cee Michaela
www.Zuleana.com

Note: Items marked with an asterisk are available for purchase on my website.

Liquids	Fruits	Veggies	Proteins	Snacks	Spices
30 Calorie Almond Milk	Apples (red or green)	Spinach Kale Bok choy Romaine Lettuce	Skinless Chicken	17 Raw Almonds per day	Organic Turmeric
Alkaline Water	Apricots Avocado	Collard Greens	Skinless Turkey	3-4 Brazil Nuts per day	Organic Ceylon Cinnamon
Beet Juice	Blueberries Blackberries Raspberries Strawberries	Turnip greens Carrots Celery Cabbage	Salmon (wild caught)	6 Olives Pomegranate Seeds	Organic Cardamom
Carrot Juice	Grapefruit Kiwi Lemon Lime 13 Cherries	Brussels Sprouts Cauliflower Asparagus Okra Zucchini	Albacore Tuna Sardines (wild caught) Herring	Sunflower Seeds **OILS** 100% MCT	Organic Ginger Powder Organic Pink Sea Salt
	Pear Red Grapes	Squash Sweet potato Butternut Squash	Mackerel Anchovy	Extra Virgin Coconut Oil Extra Virgin Olive Oil	Bragg 24 Herbs & Spices
	2 SMALL Bananas per week	Cucumbers Beets Onion Garlic Leeks Mushrooms	*Spirulina Powder *Hemp Protein	**DRESSINGS** Bragg Raspberry or Pomegranate Vinaigrette	Cracked Fresh Pepper Organic Vanilla Extract

SPECIAL DIETARY NOTE: We eat a very small bowl of watermelon (due to TOXIC LECTINS and high sugar level) only 1-2 times a week during summer months. We eat just a few (very small) pieces of pineapple (because of the sugar level) – once a week.

Coming to America

It seems like everybody wants to pack up and come to America. Hey, why not? I mean we have New York, the city that never sleeps, Philadelphia, the city of brotherly love, Vegas, the Grand Canyon, Niagara Falls, the Redwood Forest, Broadway, Hollywood, celebrities, top universities, amazing scholarships, educational fellowships, and research centers. You can have the opportunity to be an entrepreneur, own a business or buy a fabulous home. You can roll out in your cool, racy car with your top dropped, zipping down I-95 south to get your very own pair of Mickey Mouse ears at the wonderful world of Disney!

The problem with America is SAD, the Standard American Diet which is…well…SAD! I have seen many beautiful Asian women, commonly known for their svelte body types, arrive in the U.S. and within a few months are now, well, how should I say it, "abundantly blessed with extra junk in their trunks!" Yes, America's food will have you fat and sick. This food will have you feeling like you woke up on the wrong side of a bed without a mattress and then thrown under a fast-moving bus! America could you not have sent out a notice, a warning, an alert, a doggone smoke signal concerning all of these crazy GMOs in our food? What about the pesticides and toxins in our fruits and vegetables? The chemicals in the plastics? What about LECTINS? Let me stay calm and break this down for you, my fellow friends and countrymen.

GMOs are genetically modified organisms. These are foods that are *engineered and are simply FAKE.* They contain hardly any nutrients. This is a way for America to mass produce food and make mega quick money. We like to call it "FRAKENFOODS!" They are fruits that are usually larger in appearance and very shiny and beautiful. They are sometimes called conventional fruit and even have a PLU (price look up) code, consisting of four to five digits that start with the number four. In my research, I have found that if a fruit starts with a four, it's usually filled with pesticides. As the first number goes lower or down to having no number at all, you have got yourself a handy- dandy, super-tasty (NOT)...GMO! No wonder America is feeling so weak and fatigued! Can you give us some real nutrients please?

Then they spray horrible, deadly chemicals on the fruit to help protect the crops from bugs. Okay that's cool for the bugs but does your fancy spray have to kill us, too? Never fear America, they don't call me the **Harriet Tubman of Health** for nothing. I got you covered. Simply look for the PLU (price look up) code that starts with the number nine, these are the organic fruits and foods. Just remember, nine is fine.

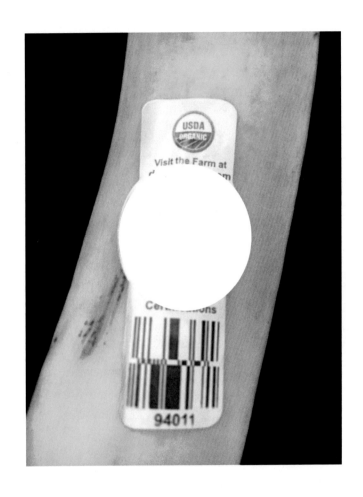

Just remember, ***nine is fine.***

Now, let's keep calm and carry on to the dangers of toxic lectins. Lectins are a certain naturally occurring protein that can cause massive damage to the digestive system. It can lead to nausea, vomiting, and even leaky gut syndrome. Lectins may cause inflammation and allergies. The following foods contain lectins: beans, wheat, dairy, soy, lentils, peanuts, peas, melons, peppers, eggplant, potatoes, tomatoes, and shell fish.

In fact, about 20% of rheumatoid arthritis cases are caused by lectins in the nightshade family, which include the following: **potatoes, tomatoes, eggplant, and bell peppers**. **Wheat**, which has a huge amount of lectins, can cause thyroid weakness. Did you know **kidney beans** become five times more toxic when heated to 80 degrees Celsius? Okay, I can hear all of you so clearly right now saying, "What the heck?! Enough is enough. This is cray-cray! I can't even!" It's okay. I got you. Don't panic. In fabulous Zuleana® style and deeply influenced by Susan Bennett, the voice of famous iPhone's "assistant," Siri, we will all simply start "RECACULATING ROUTE!" We will do our best to eat as few lectins as possible. So here we go.

HOW ZULEANA®DEALS WITH CRAY-CRAY LECTINS!

On the Zuleana® way, we will eat the following:

- 17 almonds every day
- 1 small sweet potato once a week
- 1-2 boiled, organic, cage-free pasture raised or local, farm fresh eggs one to three times a week (take out the yolk or ½ of the yolk for less fat and cholesterol if you so desire.

1 small cup of watermelon once or twice a week during summer months (no cantaloupe/honeydew)

- 1 very small tomato on our salads once or twice a week
- A few sunflower and/or pumpkin seeds twice a week
- No peppers (I know. That one is hard for some.)
- No peanuts (Yuck! They are completely contaminated.)
- No beans (They give you the farts anyway!)
- *No soy whatsoever! (#soyisnotashealthyasyouthink)*
- *N*o corn (hard to digest and possible GMOs)
- No COW'S MILK (too many hormones)

Yes, welcome to America, land of the GMOs…home of the toxins! And as if this wasn't enough to rain on our lovely Zuleana® parade, have you not noticed the missing bees? Shhhh…come closer. Let me tell you all about… ***the secret life of bees.***

The Secret Life of Bees

Bees totally rock! They are the true hustlers of all creatures on the planet. They are responsible for pollinating a third of everything that we eat such as squash, broccoli, almonds, apples, and herbs. These elements are some of the most important parts of our Zuleana® eating lifestyle. It's important to get in good with your local bee keeper. There are two problems I have found. The first is that many of them HEAT their honey, which burns away most of its vitamins and enzymes. Secondly, they have no SEEDS in their honey! You are probably totally perplexed saying, "What seeds? What in the devil are you talkin' about Coach Cee Cee?"

In the Zuleana® lifestyle we love our honey raw. Honey that has never been heated. It is unrefined and it still has the enzymes, pollen, and PROPOLIS SEEDS! Your honey should have a beautiful, light-yellow, creamy appearance and little tiny brown seeds on the top called propolis. This is also known as bee glue, which the bees use to seal holes in their hive and to protect the hive from invaders. Be sure to eat every last seed. They are tiny and tasteless and the health benefits are phenomenal.

Propolis seed benefits include the following:

- Builds your immunity, common cold, and flu
- Supports antioxidants, anti-bacterial, anti-fungal, anti-viral
- Fights acne and dermatitis, heals burns, and prevents dental cavities
- Prevents the spread of cancer and chemo side effects
- Prevents respiratory tract infection and allergies
- Eliminates the parasite giardiasis
- Helps with cold sores and genital herpes

WHOA! And guess what? I have a propolis-based healing skin cream ($3) and propolis/aloe-based (no fluoride) tooth gel ($8) on my website in the online store, so be sure to stop and shop. In the Zuleana® way, we drink (add it to our matcha tea powder) or eat (in our steel-cut oatmeal) a little honey with propolis seed every single day. The power is in the seed! I have the one pound jars of this creamy dreamy stuff ($12) at my natural product presentations. So be sure to check my events calendar. ;)

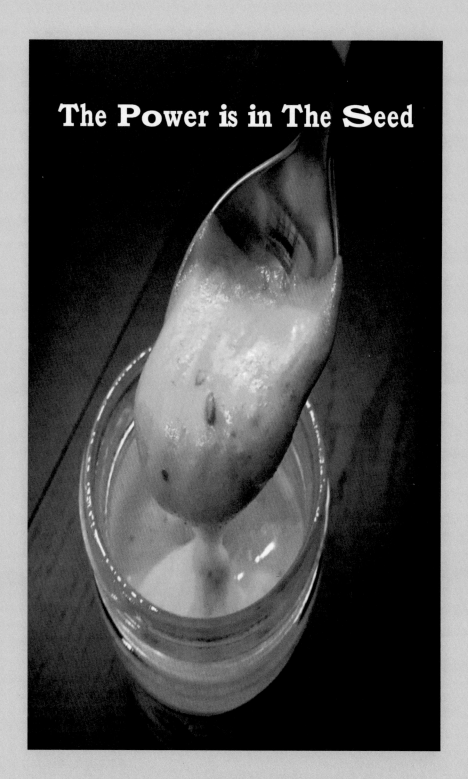

The **Power** is in The **S**eed

Why Is Your Fat Not Moving?

Have you ever noticed no matter how much you cut back on eating, no matter how much you exercise like crazy, your stubborn belly fat will not budge?! After successfully helping thousands of women lose massive amounts of weight, the following things are what I have discovered retain those pounds:

- **Weak thyroid**
- **Lack of fiber**
- **Constipation and/or a dirty colon**
- **Adrenal fatigue**
- **High cortisol and/or high stress level**
- **Lack of sleep and/or lack of exercise**
- **Sluggish liver and/or weak kidneys**
- **Dirty colon**
- **Missing gall bladder**
- **Lack of nutrients (vitamin/mineral deficiencies)**
- **Lack of portion control**
- **Eating the wrong foods**
- **Eating empty calories**
- **Water retention**

Once you start eating the Zuleana® way, the nutrients and food combinations will naturally address ALL of the above issues. So don't worry. We got this! Let me break down my famous three-piece weight loss system: **THE MELT BELLY FAT BOX.**

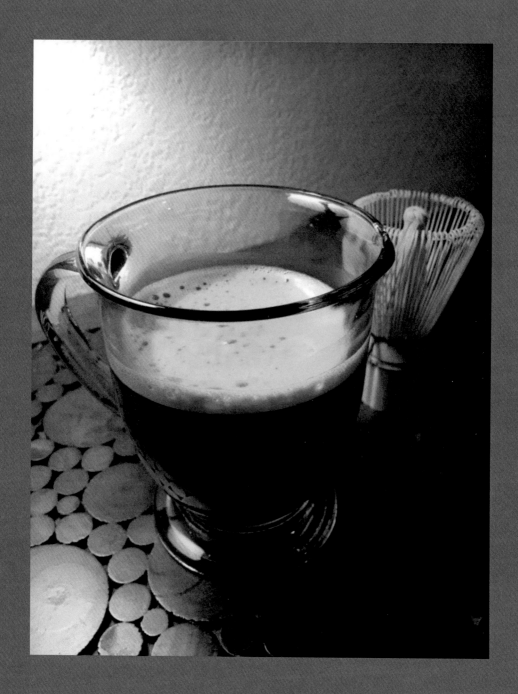

Piece 1: The Love of Matcha
THE BELLY FAT BURNER

This powerful tea powder made of finely ground green tea leaves is the absolute center of the Zuleana® lifestyle. I was drinking matcha (which I affectionately call *melt belly fat tea*...LOL), way before it was mega-popular. I began to drink it every morning with a bit of raw honey and I lost 30 pounds in three months **_without_** exercise! This tea has changed my life forever.

This is why it is the very first element in my three-piece weight loss system. The tea is from Japan and is ceremonial grade. Matcha powder has to be a very high grade and have no added fillers or sugar in order to receive all of its health benefits, which include the following:

- Melts belly fat and boost metabolism
- Cleans the brain and detoxes the body
- Helps mental focus and calmness
- Promotes better energy
- Lowers cholesterol and stabilizes blood sugar levels
- Helps reduce high blood pressure
- Lowers the risk of heart disease
- Prevents cancer

More Amazing Matcha Facts

- Matcha has 137 times more antioxidants than regular green tea.

- 1 cup of MATCHA is equivalent to drinking 10 cups of regular green tea as far as nutritional content.

- Matcha provides a mega dose of antioxidants.

- Matcha provides Vitamin C, chromium, selenium, magnesium, and zinc.

- Matcha contains a special antioxidant called catechins, which provide potent cancer fighting properties.

- Matcha contains a powerful polyphenol called EGCG (epigallo-catechin gallate). This polyphenol is known for boosting metabolism and halting the growth of cancer.

Piece 2: Artichoke Leaf Tea

THE LIVER CLEANSER

Artichoke leaf tea has a beautifully mild taste and is very healthy for the body. Artichoke leaf tea is chock-full of polyphenols and is great at cleaning the liver. The liver is the largest internal organ and is responsible for hundreds of chemical actions. For weight loss and maximum total health, the liver must be cleansed and protected. The liver is your blood purifier and breaks down your fat. Artichoke tea is very popular in Vietnam.

Here are the benefits of artichoke leaf tea:

- Protects the liver and liver function
- Helps regulate the sugars in blood
- Cleanses bad cholesterol
- Lowers blood pressure levels
- Strengthens the gallbladder
- Helps digestion, bloating, and heartburn
- Rids excess water retention
- Prevents heart diseases and strokes
- Helps IBS
- Clears the skin

Piece 3: Diatomaceous Earth
THE HEAVY METAL CLEANSER

This gentle *white powder detox* is often referred to as "DE" and has no taste. It is made of fossilized remains of marine organisms called diatoms. The powder contains lots of silica and is incredibly gentle yet highly effective in detoxifying the body. No, you will not be nursing the toilet all day. LOL! Take one heaping teaspoon of food grade DE with 8 oz. of water, preferably at night before you go to sleep. Drink DE on an empty stomach and drink water throughout the day for best results.

DE benefits include:

- Cleanses toxins from the blood and liver
- Cleanses bacteria, viruses, and yeast (candida)
- Regulates bowel movements
- Curbs gas and cleans digestive tract- **IBS**
- Reduces internal odors
- Improves bone mineralization and low bone mass (ostcoporosis)
- Protects joints and ligaments
- Grows stronger nails and teeth
- Eliminates parasites and *heavy metals

*Common heavy metals are the following: mercury, lead, aluminum, and arsenic. Heavy metals can be very toxic to the body.

How to be a Master Steeper

Many people don't steep their tea long enough to effectively infuse it. You must infuse your tea bags to get the maximum potency of your herbs. The longer a tea steeps, the greater the flavonoids. A diet rich in flavonoids is usually associated with reduced risk of heart disease, cancer, asthma, and stroke.

1. Heat up your spring or purified water and bring to a boil. Note: never use distilled or faucet water. Distilled water will leave your tea tasting flat and faucet water has too many chemicals.
2. Pour hot water over 1-2 tea bags and cover with a small plate.
3. Allow the tea bags to steep for 5-6 minutes.
4. Squeeze all the liquid out of the bag, toss the bag, and drink up.

Zuleana® note: steeping is great for all herbal teas; however, matcha green tea (powder) is best used with cool to warm water. Excessive heat kills the health properties of matcha.

Zuleana® and Diabetes

To keep your glycemic load low, blood sugar and insulin leveled properly, you must follow these Zuleana® rules.

- Do not eat watermelon, pineapple, guava, papaya, or mango.

- Do not eat artificial sugar, white/brown/raw SUGAR, AGAVE OR HONEY (not even raw honey). Do use Stevia if you have diabetes.

- Do not eat carrots. The starch turns into sugar too quickly, which spikes blood sugar.

- Do not eat brown rice. The starch turns into sugar too quickly, which spikes blood sugar.

- Do not eat beans. The starch turns into sugar too quickly, which spikes blood sugar.

- Drink/eat 1 tsp. of Ceylon cinnamon every day.

- Drink guava leaf tea every day. (Available in my online store).

- Take chromium pills daily. (Available in my online store).

- Eat only two low-glycemic fruits per day.

- Sweet potatoes can spike your blood sugar as well!

Zuleana®
Mandatory Lifestyle Rules

- Eat 1,200 calories a day.

- Every meal should contain beautiful colors.

- Exercise and burn 500 calories 5-6 days per week. Consume about 20 grams of protein after your workout. I suggest hemp protein, which contains 20 amino acids and is easy to digest.

- Rest your body on Sunday or your chosen day of rest.

- Don't skip breakfast and don't eat past 8 p.m. Skipping breakfast can increase your risk of obesity.

- Eat a boiled egg with cracked pepper, turmeric, and a dash of pink Himalayan sea salt if you get a craving during the day. You can take half of the yolk out to save calories.

- Make sure all chicken and turkey has NO HORMONES and NO ANTIBIOTICS.

- Make sure all eggs have NO HORMONES, NO ANTIBIOTICS, are CAGE FREE, and are PASTURE-RAISED/ FARM FRESH.

- Make certain all fish is WILD CAUGHT and SUSTAINABLY HARVESTED.

- Check that all fruits and veggies are ORGANIC.

- Cut out alcohol. Beer is full of sugar and wine contains sugar and estrogenic properties. Alcohol weakens the liver, the organ responsible for fat metabolism.

- Eat unsalted, raw almonds and seeds, not trail mix or dried fruits

42

- Sleep sweetly for 7-8 hours. This builds your metabolism and gives your body proper rest and recovery time.

- Read ALL labels carefully. This will help you make wiser choices concerning your calories, fat, carbs, sodium, etc.

- Make sure you measure your foods. You must get used to what one serving looks like. When making your oatmeal, be very careful to not pour oatmeal into your bowl. Don't douse dressing over your salad. A proper serving of salad dressing is one tablespoon and a serving of oatmeal is ½ cup. Measuring will help keep you on track so you don't overeat.

Note that you can add chia seeds to your oatmeal. They contain lots of fiber, omega-3 fats, calcium, iron, and protein. You can also add a bit of flaxseed (milled or ground) to your oatmeal as well, especially after menopause. Flaxseed provides fiber, improves heart health and digestive system, and lowers the risk of diabetes and cancer.

The Zuleana® Tools
A Journal

It is very important to write down your Zuleana® journey. Take notes of your calorie intake, portion size, and your mood. The more you write and study your habits and goals, the more weight or diseases you will lose. You may also see improvement in your blood work. You might even drop some medications. Write everything down because the whole process will be your journey! To actually keep a record and see your strengths and weaknesses as well as your progress will make a big difference in your success.

A Scale and A Tape Measure

You will need a scale and a tape measure. Be sure to write down your starting weight and inches of waist, arms, and thighs. Weigh yourself at least once a week. It's best to weigh yourself in the morning before you drink or eat. Many Zuleana® girls lose more inches than pounds in the beginning. *Zuleana® girls have been known to easily lose 5-10 pounds in their first week!* Whether in pounds or inches, it is exciting to watch yourself disappear!

#watchmedisappear   #Zuleanamakesyoudisappear

The Zuleana®Difference

Zuleana® is balanced in *every* area of life! We believe that toxins and hormones are causing horrific amounts of weight gain and diseases in the body. Therefore, Zuleana® focuses on using leaves, herbs, vitamins, minerals, spices, nutrients, and phytonutrients to rid the body of excess chemicals, hormones, toxins, and fat.

Zuleana® cuts out almost all *red meat and avoids processed meats and foods. Because of the dangers of synthetic hormones, we do not drink cow's milk. Instead, we drink almond milk. We concentrate on eating as many antioxidants, flavonoids, fiber and good enzymes as possible. Zuleana® builds your immune system, cleanses your liver and colon, protects your brain and other organs, balances your hormones, increases your energy, boosts your metabolism, clears your skin, and helps you obtain an overall sense of vitality and total well-being. In Zulean®, we eat, play, walk, run, swim, work, pray, breathe, rest, and get exciting results.

*We are allowed to eat 3 oz. of grass-fed lamb on occasion.

ZULEANA® SURPRISES!

In case you didn't know, a Zuleana® girl can eat the following GOOD FATS and lose massive weight.

- **Avocados (2-3 slices or 1/3 twice a week)**
- **Almonds (17 a day)**
- **Coconut oil (1-2 tbs. per day)**
- **DARK CHOCOLATE... every single day, usually at lunch time!**

   Extra Credit: The Zuleana® girls eat the dark chocolate (.375 oz.) from my website, which has 99% cacao. This means it has a super-rich taste, a low sugar content, and releases way more antioxidants with every dreamy bite. BAM!

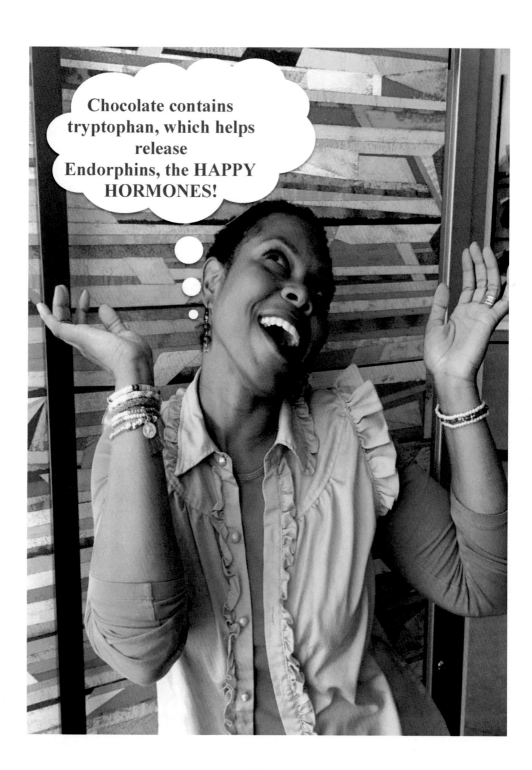

HAVE YOU EVER REALLY CONSIDERED THE HEALTH BENEFITS OF JOY?

Coach Cee Cee's Personal Observation:

When it comes to really losing weight, diet is way more important than exercise. Every food works differently in your body and you also have to confuse the body by mixing up your calorie count. Zuleana® girls might eat 1,200 calories on one day, 1,250 another, and maybe 1,150 on another day.

Your quality of food is a key factor in burning body fat successfully. Antioxidants, alkaline foods, and polyphenols will help you lose way more weight than foods that have no nutrients or that are full of sugar and fat. Herbs are very nutritious. Cilantro has about 20 health benefits in itself and fennel tea (located in my online store) is great for flatulence, stomach issues, and fibroids. Some of our favorite herbs are the following: cilantro, parsley, thyme, rosemary basil, and mint leaves. Herbs are incredibly helpful in keeping cancer at bay.

Many of the Zuleana® girls like to exercise in the morning. We exercise because we want to normalize our glucose. We have noticed that exercising at night can help the glucose level in the morning. We also exercise to get a stronger heart, a recharged mind, amazing oxygen, a better mood, keep that nasty stress away, and improve our libidos. Whoop! Whoop!

SECRET #1:
Sweet Sleep

You are not a night owl. You are a human being! Please go to sleep for seven to eight hours every night to allow for *body restoration*. Try to go to bed at the same time every night in order to regulate your sleep pattern and turn off ALL the lights (including the TV and technology) for maximum melatonin production. Melatonin is a hormone that the brain produces. It maintains your circadian rhythm (sleep-wake cycle). It is also known to prevent cancer and help those with menopause, depression, heart disease, fibromyalgia, pain, and even children with autism.

Don't forget to eat dinner foods that are filled with serotonin (our sleep-promoting hormone) no later than 8p.m. You should always give your digestive system about three hours to *work it all out* before you hit the sack. A perfect ZULEANA® serotonin meal would consist of turkey, brown rice, and spinach or a spinach salad with egg whites and quinoa.

Zuleana® Girls Have Alkaline Bodies

Your body is either acidic or alkaline. A body that is acidic will be prone to fat and disease while an alkaline body will usually be more lean, healthy, and disease-free. Alkaline is more than just fancy water. There are many foods that are alkaline as well. Alkaline foods are incredibly nutrient-dense. They nourish and energize your cells, which helps to build more *mithochondria!*

Zuleana® Top Alkaline Foods:

- **Alkaline water**
- **Almonds and brazil nuts**
- **Avocados**
- **Quinoa**
- **Grasses such as wheatgrass**
- **Green veggies–spinach, kale, collards, cabbage, romaine lettuce, mustard greens**
- **Miso**
- **Sweet potatoes**
- **Seaweed**
- **Stevia (a sweetener)**
- **Lemon, lime, and grapefruit**

Zuleana® Girls Love Antioxidants

There is a process called oxidative stress, which cause free radicals to run rampant through the body, attack the cells, and possibly cause cancer. These free radicals cause the cells to age and not function properly. Free radicals come from toxins so unfortunately we all have them. An antioxidant is any food that fights oxidative stress. That is why it is called an *ANTI*-oxidant. So the more of them that you consume, the more your cells will be healthy and energized.

ZULEANA® TOP ANTIOXIDANT FOODS LIST

- Dark chocolate
- Wild blueberries
- Blackberries
- Cilantro
- Cinnamon
- Oregano
- Turmeric
- Basil
- Ginger
- Thyme

Zuleana® Calories

In the Zuleana® way, we eat 1,200 calories per day.

You can break those calories up. Here is an example:

breakfast: 200 cal.   lunch: 400 cal.

dinner: 400 cal.   snacks: 200 cal.

POPULAR ZULEANA®FOODS CALORIE LIST

- ½ bowl of **gluten-free**, steel-cut oatmeal: 150 calories

- ½ cup of blue berries: 41 calories

- 1 small apple: 78 calories

- ½ grapefruit: 50 calories

- 1 banana: 105 calories

- 17 almonds: 100 calories

- 1 boiled egg: 78 calories

- 4 oz. chicken: 187 calories

- 4 oz. turkey: 200 cal. dark/158 cal. white meat

- 4 oz. salmon: grilled 200 cal./ baked- 185 cal.

- 4 oz. tuna: 209 calories

- 13 cherries: 52 calories

- 20 red grapes: 60 calories

- ½ cup of brown rice: 150 calories

- ½ cup of spinach: 23 calories

Zuleana® Proteins

As females, we only need about 50 grams of proteins per day and that is if we live a sedentary life. So, in the Zuleana® way, once we eat 4 oz. of chicken (35 grams of protein) and 4 oz. of wild caught salmon (23 grams of protein) in a given day, that's already a total of 58 grams of protein.

We also try to exercise 5 to 6 days a week to burn 500 calories a day. So when we exercise, I like to make sure we get about 75-100 grams of protein per day, which can easily be obtained by adding spirulina and/or my favorite greens powder, Vitamineral Green™ by HealthForce (both are available on my website) to your matcha powder in the morning. Steel-cut oatmeal yields 5 grams of protein and your snack bag of raw almonds yield 6 grams. So your protein count can add up pretty quickly. Protein helps the body build muscle and gives you proper energy. We do not do a lot of protein shakes or bars as they usually contain soy, whey, and other harmful additives.

Zuleana® Carbs

Zuleana® girls eat **nutrient-dense CARBS** that help us lose weight and maintain our energy.

- Gluten-free oatmeal blasts visceral fat and provides 27 grams of carbs per ½ cup serving.

- Quinoa is the super protein! It has all 9 essential amino acids and builds lean muscle and revs up the metabolism. It contains 20 grams of carbs per ½ cup serving.

- Vegetables provide fiber, vitamins, minerals, and antioxidants, for example, a sweet potatoes contains 27 grams of carbs.

- Brown rice provides slow-burning fiber, essential vitamins, magnesium, and vitamin B6. It contains 34 grams of carbs per ½ cup serving.

- Pear (small)–27 grams of carbs

- Apple (small)–25 grams of carbs

Note that we need about 40-50 grams of carbs a day to stay super healthy and lean…the Zuleana® way. We must work out to help burn the carb count.

Zuleana® Thyroid Care

I always suggest that each lady be proactive in self-care and start strengthening her thyroid immediately as this is the gland that regulates the body temperature and metabolism. It also controls heart rate.

Here is an underactive thyroid check:

- Cold hands and feet
- Very dry skin and hair
- Headaches
- Constipation
- Inability to sweat
- Infertility
- No desire for sex
- Permanent heel cracks
- Loss of outer third of eyebrow hair

Here are some helpful tips to strengthen your thyroid:

- Use ashwagandha to lower cortisol.

- Remove silver fillings–use a DAMS mercury safe dentist.

- Go gluten free–for example, gluten-free oatmeal).

- Use kelp and other seaweeds to raise your iodine level.

- Do a heavy metal detox using DE and turmeric pills.

- Consume more selenium such as Brazil nuts, salmon, mushroom, and onions.

- Lower intake of sugar and grains and up your good fats: avocado, wild salmon, coconut oil, hemp seed, extra virgin olive oil, and coconut milk (45 calories)

- Eat more tyrosine-filled foods such as pumpkin seeds, almonds, and avocado.

- Make sure vitamin D3 level is at 60.

SPICE GIRL NOTE
Ceylon Cinnamon

Try to buy as many organic items as you can. Organic is better quality, more nutrients, and less toxins. Yes, all of your spices should be organic, especially since you will be drinking them directly. Remember, your cinnamon must be organic Ceylon cinnamon from Sri Lanka as it is the true medicinal cinnamon. It helps with cholesterol, blood sugar level, regulates insulin, gets rid of yeast and helps with pain. Be careful with cinnamon if you have liver problems. Otherwise, swallow up to one teaspoon per day. The Ceylon cinnamon is available in my online store.

The Power of Turmeric

MELLOW YELLOW!

One of the most medicinal spices ever created is this wonderful yellow spice from India. In Zuleana®, we drink and eat a lot of turmeric. It is a main staple in our eating lifestyle and is an absolute must have and must do! There really is no limit on the daily consumption of this powerhouse spice. So feel free to add ½ teaspoon to your matcha in the morning. Add another ½ teaspoon to your brown rice or cauliflower rice. Shake it on your boiled egg or add it to dressing for your salad. You can also mix it into your wild caught tuna or dust your salmon or veggies with this powerful golden treasure. It has a unique taste that you will learn to love. You can also buy the turmeric/bromelain capsules (for major pain issues) from my online store.

The benefits of turmeric are the following:

- Inflammation and joint pain
- Brain health
- Liver cleanse
- Cancer prevention
- Lupus and fibromyalgia

Note that you can take the turmeric capsules and eat or drink the turmeric at the same time. It is actually even more powerful when you do both. **Be sure to swallow turmeric pills with good fat such as almond milk, chicken, turkey, salmon.**

Ashwagandha Is Our Bestie

This amazing adaptogenic herb is very popular in Ayurvedic (holistic healing methods from India) medicine and has all of our favorite girlie-girl benefits.

- Lowers cortisol

- Helps sluggish thyroid

- Relieves stress

- Protects the brain

- Improves Alzheimer's

- Alleviates depression

- Takes away anxiety

- Improves your mood and energy

- Boost immunity

- Helps adrenal fatigue

- **BALANCES HORMONES!** (Okay, you can go ahead and do your happy dance now.)

Note that ashwagandha capsules are available on my website.

GOLDEN INDIAN MILK

TURWAGANDA

Turmeric + Ashwagandha = heavenly drink

1. Heat 1 cup of almond milk and ½ tbs. of coconut oil.

2. Add 1 tbs. of raw honey, ¼ teaspoon each of organic turmeric, Ceylon cinnamon, organic ginger spice, organic cardamom, a dash of black pepper, and a few drops of organic Madagascar vanilla flavoring.

3. Open 1 ashwagandha capsule (300 mg) and pour the powder into the mixture.

4. Use a bamboo whisk and bowl or blend in a blender.

You can drink it hot or add ice and drink it cold. When you heat up the almond milk and add turmeric, it increases the solubility of curcumin, which is part of turmeric. The piperine found in black pepper when mixed with turmeric greatly increases the absorption of turmeric in the body.

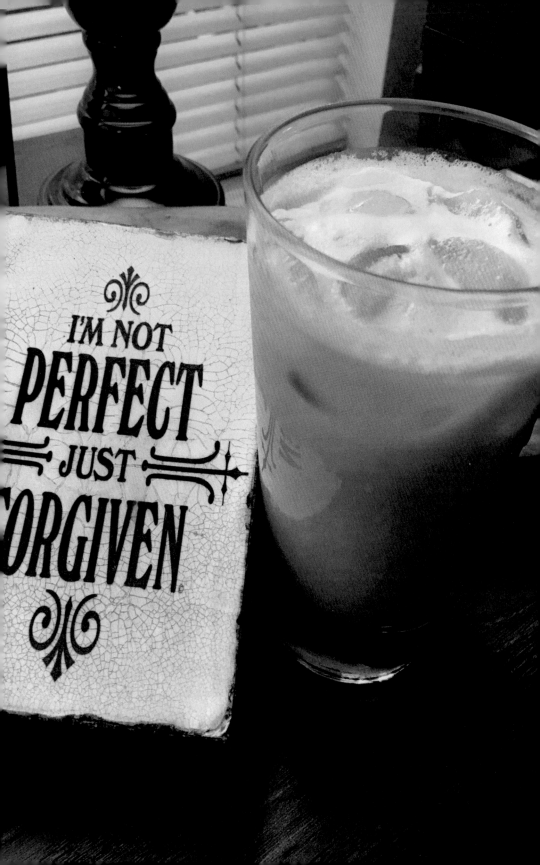

SECRET #2:
Craving Endorphins

Zuleana® Girls Smile

Smiling actually releases endorphins. The more this *happy hormone* releases in your body, the better you will feel. *Depression cannot live in a body that is constantly releasing endorphins!* Did you know when you smile, the facial muscles stretch and trigger the brain to produce endorphins, which produces feelings of happiness? Wow. Go, God!

Zuleana® Girls Laugh

Children are known to laugh approximately 300 times a day as opposed to adults who laugh only 5 times a day. SMH! Laughter helps produce endorphins. So let's all begin to laugh again.

Zuleana® Girls Cry

When we break down and cry, the tension builds, the tears flow, and then the body feels a release and produces endorphins. So cry, baby, cry!

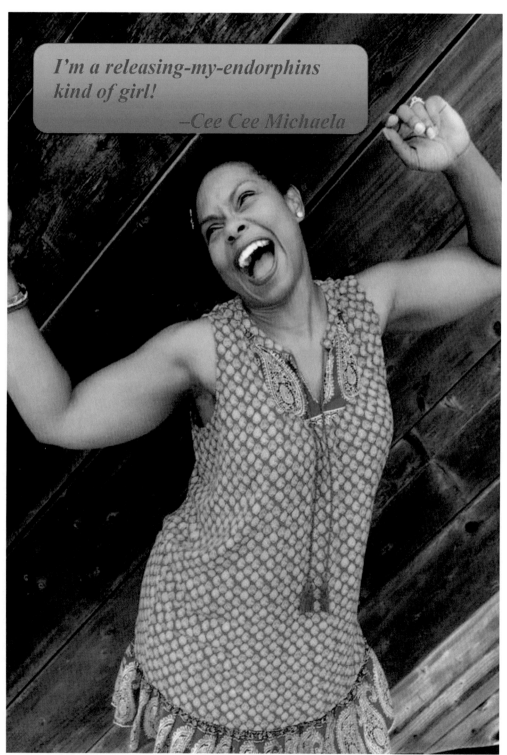

Other Ways to Release Endorphins

- Sniff the scent of vanilla or lavender
- Exercise
- Listen to music
- Take a little ginseng
- Eat spicy food
- Kissing or sex
- Eat 70-99% dark chocolate

OMG! Okay, there goes that dark chocolate again. Research shows that dark chocolate provides protection against heart attacks and stroke. Its high content of polyphenols and antioxidants reduces inflammation, lowers blood pressure, reduces bad cholesterol, raises good cholesterol, and protects arteries.

Endorphins are natural pain killers!

Just think, all we have to do is smile or be filled with laughter. Like the Bible says in Proverbs 17:22: "A merry heart does good like a medicine, but a broken spirit dries the bones!"

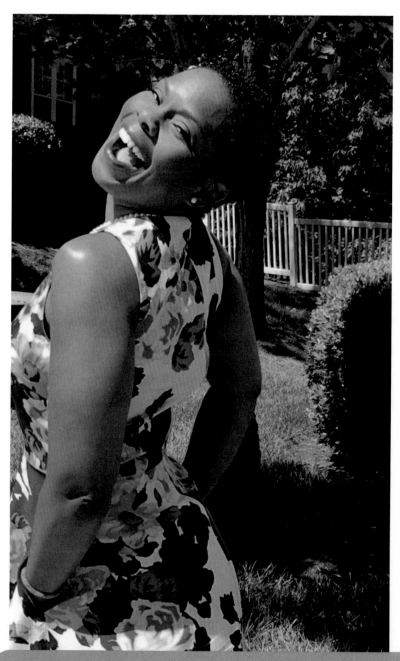

Don't let anyone break your spirit, chile!
—Cee Cee Michaela

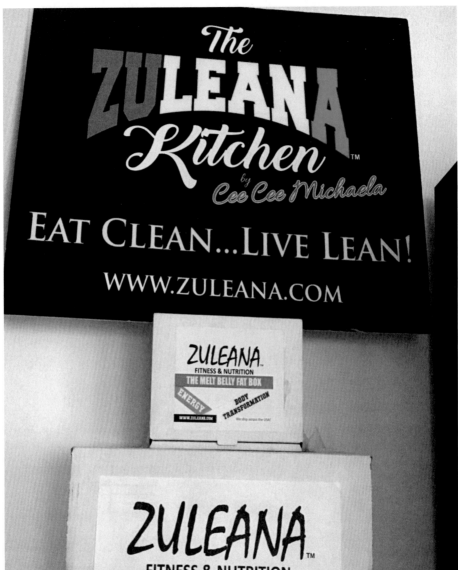

The Biggest Zuleana® Eating Lifestyle MISHAPS!

- Leaving skin on your meats.
- Eating dark meat which has more fat.
- Eating too many olives or capers because they are very salty. We are allowed 6 olives per serving, per day.
- Not eating a bit of fermented organic sauerkraut for gut health.
- Not taking a 50 billion CFU probiotic, which helps the gut.
- Not measuring salad dressing.
- Eating beans…a BIG NO-NO.
- Eating too many proteins or carbs in one sitting.
- Cooking food in aluminum foil.
- Eating fried eggs over boiled egg–such a huge NO-NO!
- Eating too many omelets instead of oatmeal with berries in the morning.
- Not having daily bowel movements.
- Not drinking enough water–at least 12-14 (8 oz.) glasses per day or drinking ½ of your body weight in ounces.
- Cooking turkey burgers in a frying pan, which causes more grease. Instead, cook them on an indoor grill with a drip tray.
- Eating a random amount of nuts instead of simply eating 17 almonds and 3 to 4 Brazil nuts, daily.
- Only consuming 1 to 2 pieces of the 3-piece weight loss system! Each piece cleanses and strengthens different organs to make weight loss and disease prevention successful.
- Allowing negative surprises or stressful situations to overtake the wiser and healthier choice to eat clean and exercise.

SECRET #3:

Long Life

Here are my top 9 elements that I would want every human being to consume in order to be healthy, vibrant, and live to be 100 years of age or longer:

- **Matcha green tea**
- **Turmeric**
- **Raw honey**
- **Ceylon cinnamon**
- **Coconut oil**
- **Spirulina**
- **Onions**
- **Garlic**
- **Vitamin D3 capsules (available in my online store)**

    Note: I make sure my D3 does not contain the harmful ingredient, titanium dioxide .

    In the Zuleana® way, we try to consume these elements on a daily basis for a vibrant, *long life*!

SELF-CARE CHECKLIST

- Yearly gynecologist exam

- Pap smear every 3 years

- Thyroid checked by age 30

- Mammogram by age 40

- Colonoscopy by age 50

- 25-hydroxy Vitamin D every year (especially for African Americans who are at risk)–**Vitamin D3**

- Blood type test (try to remember it)

- Vitamin B12 test (esp. by age 60)–Symptoms include: dizziness, a pins and needles feeling or numbness, pale complexion, forgetfulness, unexplained fatigue, blurred or double vision, and/or muscle weakness

- Yearly eye exam

- Dental cleaning every 6 months

- Prostate exam by age 40, not 50

50 SHADES of WHITE!

In the Zuleana® eating lifestyle, we stay away from several "*dangerous-to-your-health*" white items which are the following:

- Sugar
- Salt (We do use pink sea salt. ½ teaspoon per day is the limit)
- Flour
- Pasta
- Crackers
- Sour cream
- Cream of wheat
- Grits
- Whipped cream
- Whip topping
- Mayonnaise
- White potatoes (including red skin potatoes)
- Yogurt and ice cream
- Cow's milk (We drink 30 calorie almond milk.)
- Whey and soy
- Blue cheese and all cheeses except a bit (1 oz.) of feta and/or goat cheese. **Note that 1 oz. is the size of a domino.**

Note that conventional cow's milk creates mucus and mucus creates inflammation. And contrary to what you may believe, most yogurts are filled with sugars and additives and cause gut irritation.

SMASH-T

This is an acronym for the types of fish we eat.

- Salmon

- Mackerel

- Anchovy

- Sardines (wild caught)

- Herring

- Tuna (wild caught albacore- usually in a pack, not a can)

These fish are all super high in omega-3, which is great for the brain and pain. We do not eat many bottom feeders at all and the above fish simply have more nutrients. Almost all tilapia is completely contaminated. Be sure to buy fresh, wild caught, and sustainably harvested fish for less mercury contamination.

The Power of Spirulina

Spirulina is a blue-green algae and is one of the most potent foods on the planet. In my opinion, it is one of the greatest protein sources (gram for gram), of many foods. It will boost your iron level and is filled with vitamin B6. Vitamin B6 is great for brain health. It is rich in vitamins A, B1, B2, B6, E and K. Vitamin A is good for longevity. Zuleana® girls add 2 teaspoons of spirulina to our matcha powder in the morning to allow these vitamins to absorb into our bodies. It feels so good to drink vitamins and minerals.

Spirulina has all 8 essential amino acids and 18 amino acids. It triggers leptin (unlike lectins), which helps with appetite control and cravings. Yay! Last but not least, spirulina produces more **stem cells**...whoa! Everybody could use more cells. When your body produces stem cells, then you have the ability, when in need of more cells, to be **REBUILT**. God is so good! Spirulina is available in my online store on my website.

The Importance of a Daily Probiotic

It would be my desire that every human being take a great probiotic every day. There is not one day that goes by that I don't take my favorite probiotic capsule which has 50 billion CFUs (colony-forming units) of good bacteria and 16 strains. (It's located in my online store.) Losing weight starts with great gut health. Adding more good bacteria will make losing weight so much easier. The millions of bacteria that live in our gut play a huge role in the way we *store fat,* balance sugar, and release hormones that make us feel full or hungry.

Make sure you take a probiotic that contains billions of good bacteria because many of them get lost in the traveling process and only a few million actually reach the gut where you need it the most. I also encourage Zuleana® girls to eat about 2 tablespoons of sauerkraut with dinner as sauerkraut is fermented and provides probiotics as well. Probiotics are very helpful for IBS, IBD, allergies, eczema, and respiratory issues.

Note that *pre*biotics are very important as well. They act as food and help to feed the probiotics. Our sources of prebiotics come from raw garlic, raw leeks, raw onions, cooked onions, asparagus, and raw bananas.

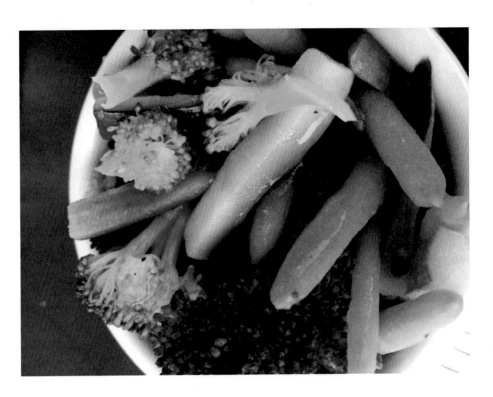

In Zuleana®, you are what you eat and what you don't eat!

Zuleana® girls learn quickly that every food choice I present to them is an element that will heal their body or greatly enhance their level of nutrients. We have no time to dwell on foods that we didn't like when we were growing up. We have to mature quickly and realize that some foods are packed with a multitude of healing properties. You must forget about your unlearned past and look forward to your new-found knowledge of healthy foods that you may have neglected and kept away from your body for so long. You have to be reprogrammed to desire that which is totally healing and healthy for your body. You must let go of unhealthy, emotionally attached and/or addictive foods.

Depression...You Must Go!

So many women are either depressed and don't even know it or they don't want to tell anyone about it. Here's how you can eat your way out of depression.

- **Salmon**
- **Oats**
- **Brazil Nuts and seeds**
- **Quinoa**
- **Cabbage**
- **Dark chocolate**
- **Sweet potatoes**
- **Kiwi**
- **Oranges**
- **Melons (may contain lectins)**
- **Apricots**
- **Natural Vitality Natural Calm (my favorite brand of magnesium)**

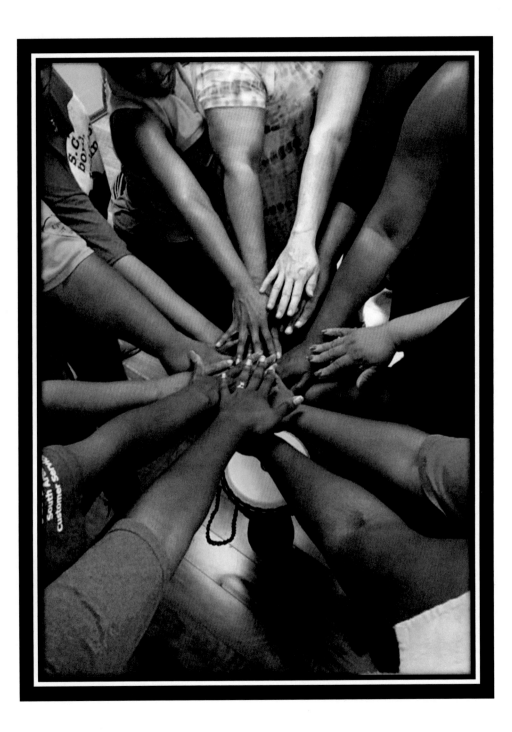

Zuleana® Poem #2: Together

God is no respecter of persons

If He can do it for me, He will do it for you

What we need in the world today is togetherness

Synergy is paramount

Isolation is a killer and you are not alone

Trust must be restored

Throwing away all competition with one another

Promises kept, solutions found

And loyalty exercised at the highest level

Be proactive, not reactive

Because we are victors not victims

We are all human and we must practice more

Understanding of one another

Placing her shoes on your feet and your sand in her

Shoes and in that moment…stop!

Listen and realize that empathy is the key

Love yourself, invest in other, and let us move forward

Pressing… persevering

Enduring

Together

The Wonders of Water

Before Step 1: Matcha

It's always good to wake up and drink a cup of warm water squeezed with ½ organic lemon and/or lime. This will help to detox your body. Then, drink about 10-12 glasses of water throughout the day. The matcha powder (step 1) and artichoke leaf tea (step 2) have a bit of caffeine so you will want to drink lots of water to stay hydrated. The water that you drink throughout the day makes your white DE powder (step 3) work exceptionally well. Water helps to hydrate the body and will help clear your skin and grow your hair. It is good to drink alkaline (9.0) water, but be sure to switch to natural spring water as well. This will ensure that you obtain naturally occurring minerals. Please be aware that many faucet filters still allow chemicals like fluoride. **Fluoride can weaken the thyroid.**

SECRET #4: Place a few cilantro leaves in your water (a crazy-good cleansing combo)!

SECRET #5: Drink 8 oz. of water before going to bed to prevent heart attacks or strokes, which usually happen during the night.

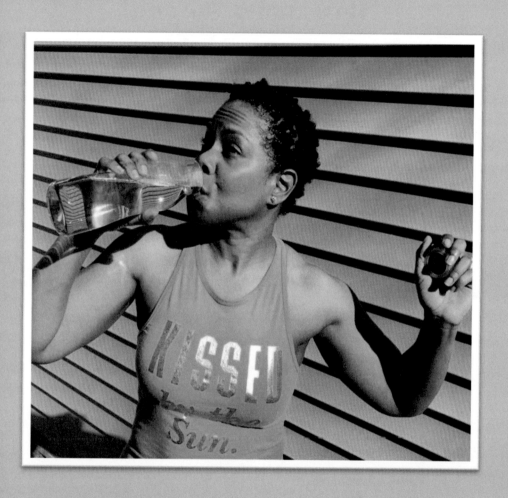

The Importance of Vitamin D3

Here comes the sun!

So many people have low Vitamin D3 levels. This affects your body in a number of negative ways. It is a fact that many African Americans are extremely low because of their darker skin pigmentation. Furthermore, the darker and/or larger a person is, the more Vitamin D3 she/he will need to obtain maximum health. Sometimes the vitamin gets trapped in the fat and does not get to the cells. A Vitamin D3 *level of 17 or below could be fatal.* Try to get your Vitamin D3 level up to a 60. This vitamin helps maintain healthy bones and teeth and reduces the risk of developing type 1 diabetes, multiple sclerosis, and breast cancer.

Here are the following symptoms of Vitamin D3 deficiency:

- **Weight gain**
- **Fatigue**
- **Cancer and cysts**
- **Depression**
- **Muscle weakness**
- **Bone pain (mild to throbbing)**
- **Head sweating**
- **Gut trouble –Crohn's, IBD, celiac, etc.**
- **Weak thyroid or thyroid nodules**

Although Vitamin D3 comes from the sun, it is best to boost your vitamin supplementation by taking a 5,000 IU (international unit) capsule, which is available from the online store on my website. **NOTE: DO NOT TAKE VITAMIN D3 ON AN EMPTY STOMACH AS IT WILL NOT PROPERLY ABSORB. Because it is a fat-soluble vitamin, it is best taken with a bit of good fat (turkey/avocado/eggs/etc.).**

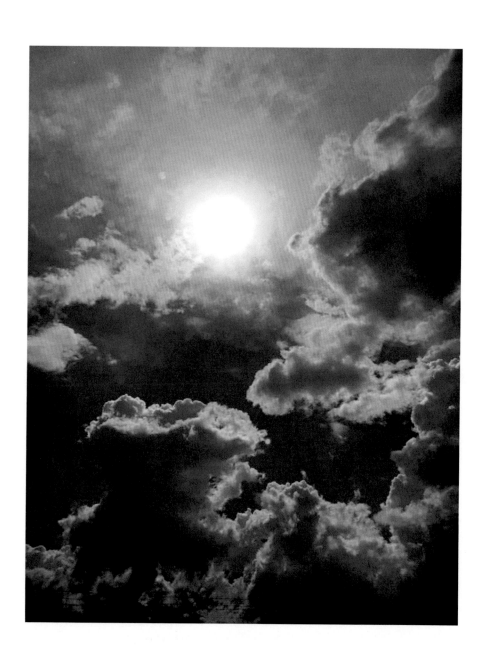

The sun shines on the just and the unjust.
Matthew 5:45

Help!
I Have a Zinc Deficiency!

Zinc is an essential mineral that is very important to the body. Women need about 8 milligrams per day. It is responsible for major brain functions, attention span, increased fertility, heart health, and immune function. Here are the following ways to know that you have a zinc deficiency:

- White lines on your nails
- Little cracks behind your ears
- Thinning hair
- Your food tastes really funny/strange
- Poor wound healing
- Nerve dysfunction
- Digestive problems/stomach-acid issues and chronic fatigue
- Thyroid nodules

Solution: Try eating zinc foods such as lamb, pumpkin seeds, chicken, turkey, eggs, mushrooms, and salmon.

Help!
My Magnesium Level is Low!

Research shows that more than (70% of women and 80% of men) do not get enough magnesium, which is responsible for over 300 bio chemical reactions in the body. My favorite magnesium (Calm) can be found in my online store and it tastes like raspberry lemonade. Oh, yeah!

Here are the symptoms of low magnesium:

- Insomnia
- Stress
- Cramps
- PMS
- Constipation
- Restless Leg Syndrome
- Anxiety
- Nervousness
- Headaches

Dangers of Estrogenic Foods

Fibroids and Tumors and Cysts...oh my!

Estrogenic foods are a danger in the Zuleana® way! They destroy your hormone balance. Fibroids are usually a build-up of mostly excess tissue and estrogen. Many estrogenic foods are what is contributing to this overly-feminized madness. They can contribute to breast cancer, **fibroids**, hypothyroidism, endometriosis, and PCOS. Stay away from the following:

- **Soy**
- **Sugar**
- **Flaxseeds (especially if you are not in or past menopause or if you already have existing womb issues)**
- **Conventional meat**
- **Conventional dairy**
- **BPA plastic and Teflon pans**
- **Birth control pills (If you are single/unmarried, try to practice abstinence.)**

To detox estrogen out of your body eat more kale, cauliflower, collard greens, broccoli, quinoa, brown rice, and *Ojibwa* cleansing tea (online store).

Help For Fibroids

- Stop eating red meat, especially beef and ham.
- Stop eating non-organic meats and processed breakfast sausages which usually have added chemicals.
- Drink less alcohol, which encourages hormonal imbalance.
- Stop eating sugar. **Sugar feeds tumors!**
- **Cook your oatmeal on the stove. Do not use instant hot cereals. Processed grains cause a sharp rise in insulin.**
- Stop drinking sodas and coffee (CAFFEINE GROWS TUMORS!)
- Stay away from cow's milk and CHEESE. They are filled with steroids and chemicals that alter your hormones and can grow fibroids.
- Stop rubbing parabens and other chemicals on your skin, especially on the belly area.
- Eat more green vegetables such as broccoli, cabbage, apples, kale, and spinach. Also include carrots and a bit of sweet potato.
- Exercise as much as possible.
- Use all natural, unbleached sanitary napkins, organic lotions, and mineral makeup. CHEMICALS cause fibroids.
- **BEWARE:** If getting fibroids removed, ask your doctor if he or she will be using the ***power morcellator,*** which breaks uterine fibroids into small pieces. **There was an FDA warning against its use.** You can research this further.
- Try *Vitex-(400-500mg twice/daily), Fish oil (1,000 mg daily), B-complex (50 mg daily), and *Ojibwa tea.
  *Items can be found in my online store.

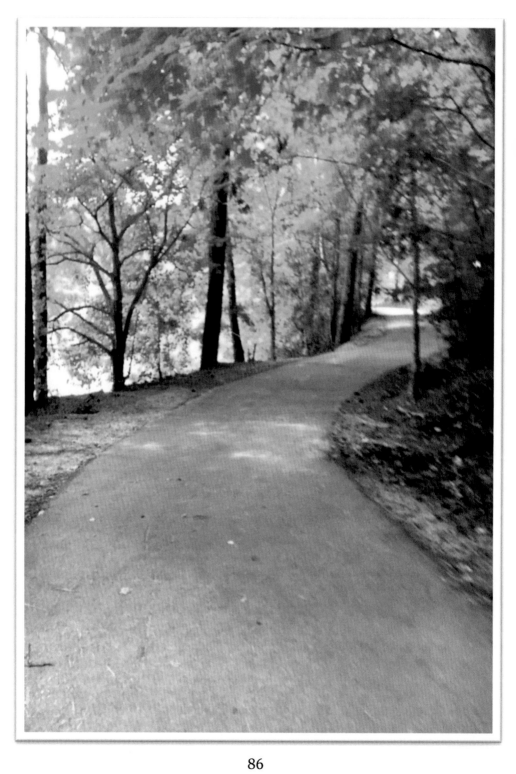

Walking

In the beginning, I encourage the Zuleana® girls to start by simply walking. Try to walk at least 30 minutes every day. Get out and enjoy all the beauty that God created just for you. There is nothing sweeter than a walking trail. The little hills, dips, and bends provide more of a challenge. A trail can boosts your spirits and sharpen your mind. You might even meet some new friends along the way.

Smile as another walker passes you. The walker will usually smile back–it's a *trail-walker* thing. I consider this gesture a little moment shared to remind us that we are all in this together and blessed to be able to walk among such natural beauty. Sometimes a simple smile is all you need to keep you moving forward. Continue on your journey and fill your lungs with fresh air. Let the trees cover you as the wind blows though the leaves and provide you with a sweet conversation saying, **"YOU CAN DO THIS!"**

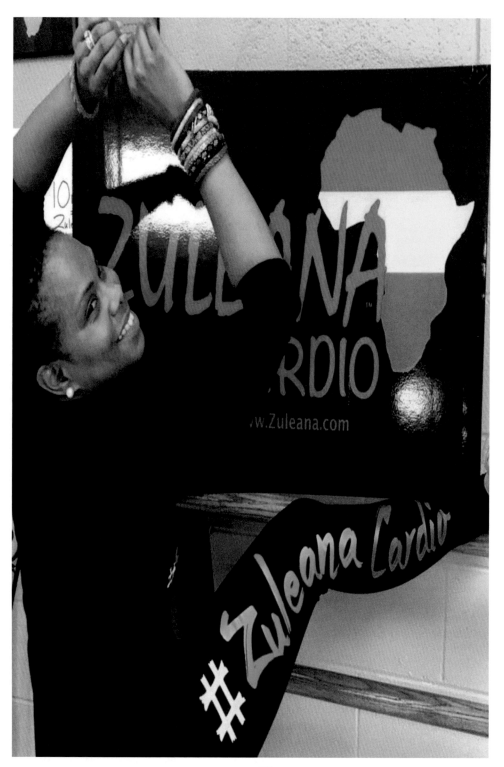

Zuleana® African Cardio

While I was living in Greenville, South Carolina, I opened my own business, Michaela's Creativity Studio LLC. It was in this beautiful place where I was blessed to teach hundreds of women about my Zuleana® brand: the colors, the style, the 3-piece weight loss system, and my weight loss dance cardio technique which all are important components of Zuleana™. Yes, dance and fitness is part of the Zuleana® lifestyle. I incorporated what I had learned many years ago during a production with the all-male acapella singing group, Ladysmith Black Mambazo. They are from South Africa and are a four-time Grammy, Award-winning collaborative phenomenon.

After performing with them, I fell in love with the Zulu culture and it stayed with me all these years. I combined my modern dance training, African dance, and Bob Fosse Broadway dance experience together to create *Zuleana® African Dance Cardio.* I have been invited to present Zuleana® to women all across the US. It's cool to be able to keynote speak and then have fun with the crowd with a cardio demo. I have had the opportunity to teach *Zuleana®*

Cardio at Furman University and Clemson University in South Carolina. I love presenting pop up events at various corporations to motivate employees with something educational, fun, and unique.

Zuleana® Cardio has a tendency to shift the entire atmosphere with feel-good vibes. The participants get to learn different moves from Africa and the music is amazing. I bring my djembe drums and shakaree. As the women gather in a circle, play the instruments, and move to the rhythm, something truly magical happens. They end up having so much fun that they forget that they are exercising! Besides, who doesn't love djembe drums and circling up with women who want to release their secret *warrior* woman?

- #zuleanawarrior
- #zuluwarrior
- #melybellyfat
- #ceeceemichaela
- #zuleanacardio
- #zuleana

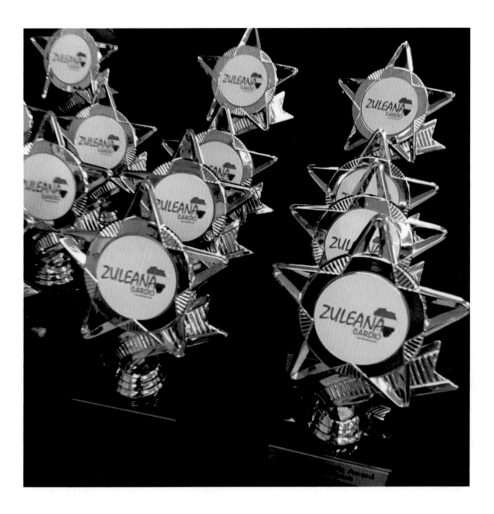

Who gives away awards to women for dropping pounds and diseases with the Zuleana® Weight Loss and Nutrition System? I do!

The Zuleana® Award

by Cee Cee Michaela

 # beagiver   #lovegives

Zuleana® Exercise Tips

I encourage those on the Zuleana® way to exercise until they burn 500 calories a day. We usually like to exercise 5-6 days a week to effectively burn the fat, boost our cardio, strengthen our muscles, and tone our bodies. You can split up the calories throughout the day if you'd like. I suggest you knock out all 500 calories first thing in the morning. It's an incredible feeling. Chances are, you might exercise again during lunch or after dinner. Here are a few tips:

- Walk in your neighborhood and chose a path that has a few small hills or maybe even a big hill. It's good to walk on an incline because it builds different muscles in your calves, thighs and glutes.
- If you have a lot of inflammation, try walking laps in a pool. You can also jog in place. Try to do some underwater bike pedaling moves and do scissors with your legs as well as underwater arm circles. The water resistance conditions the muscles and the water is easy on the joints.
- Sign up for a water aerobics or pool aquatic exercise class.
- Place your home treadmill on an incline and gradually increase your speed. Slow down and then speed up again. Be sure to interchange from flat (level 1) to incline movement (levels 6-15). Walking on an incline burns more calories and creates long, lean calf muscles.

- Buy a jump rope and get to jumping. You can burn 11 calories per minute! That is incredible.
- Perfect your hula hooping skills.
- Buy some weighted gloves and wear them during your walks. Be sure to pump your arms. You should not be able to talk when you are walking, so I am talking about a very brisk walk to a *power walk/jog-type-of-movement.*
- Walk for a few minutes, then jog, then run. Break up your pattern so that your body/muscles don't get use to the same old workout.
- Buy a kettlebell and do kettlebell swings. It works your upper body, lower body, and core. You could burn up to 400 calories in 20 minutes.
- Buy 3-8 pound free weights and start doing simple arm circles and bicep curls.
- Do 50-100 jumping jacks.
- Do 20, 50, or 100 sit ups.
- Learn how to do a plank. It is one of the most powerful and effective fitness moves ever. This no-equipment-needed move will tighten your belly, chest, arms, glutes, back, and your legs too!

Note that you do not have to eat your oatmeal before you work out if you choose to work out early in the morning. You can eat a small piece of fruit and then go work out. Just be sure to get your oatmeal with blueberries and almonds (for protein) as soon as you finish your morning workout. If you work out later in the day, be sure to eat about 30 minutes after your workout and be certain to eat some healthy, clean protein.

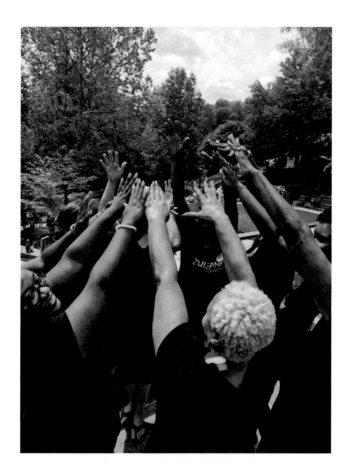

UNITY

Many ladies love my teachings and small group coaching. My Zuleana® Nutrition and Disease Prevention Conferences are held across the U.S. Go Greenville, SC, Charleston, Atlanta, Raleigh, Fayetteville, North Carolina, Maryland, Florida, Alabama, Kenner, Louisiana, Virginia, Indiana, Chicago, Arizona, Pennsylvania, and New York. You can be a Zuleana® girl too!

#Zuleanagirlzrock   #thebestisyettocome

BEFORE AND AFTERS

Let's take a moment to pause, drum roll, and reveal our **Zuleana® Biggest Winners.** They dropped it like it was hot and cold, honey! We say **"drop pounds"** in the Zuleana® way because if you **lose** weight, you just might find it again and we are **not** having that!

DRUM ROLL PLEASE...

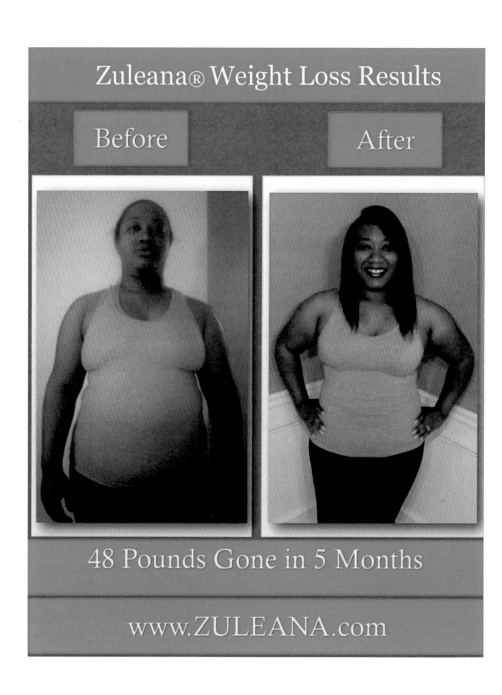

Zuleana® Weight Loss Results

Before

After

48 Pounds Gone in 5 Months

www.ZULEANA.com

Zuleana® Weight Loss Results

Before

After

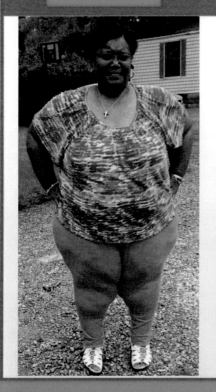
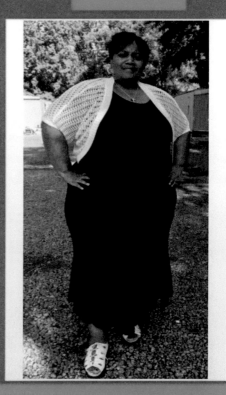

62 Pounds Gone in 77 Days

www.ZULEANA.com

TESTIMONY TIME

Some of my favorite moments were at my former studio. We would sit and have what we call, *talk time,* at the end of Zuleana® nutrition and cardio class. It would go something like this:

Testimony #1

Student: Hey, coach. I have a testimony!

Me: Awesome, let's hear it.

(Student says nothing. She simply crosses her legs over and over again.)

Me: (perplexed) What do you have to say?

Student: Ms. Cee Cee, I can cross my legs now. I have never been able to do that before Zuleana®!

(The whole class screams, hollers, rings the cow bell, and plays the djembe in excitement.)

Testimony #2

Student: Coach, I have a testimony.

Me: Sure babe, go right ahead.

Student: Look at my shoes! My strings are tied and the bow is in the middle!

Me: Sis, what do you mean?

Student: Coach, don't you know that big girls tie their shoestrings to the side?

Another student chimes in: Yeah, I use to wear loafers all the time but I can wear lace up tennis shoes now, Coach Cee Cee!

I could not believe what I was hearing. These women were being completely open and honest with me. I had always tried my best to make sure that every Zuleana® class was a safe haven where each woman could let her hair down and be herself. But in this moment, I simply broke. Tears filled my eyes and an abundance of joy filled my heart. It was in this moment that I knew-that I knew-that I knew…Zuleana® would be an international life-changing movement for all those who partake of it! These were my beautiful sisters and I was unaware of the depth of pain, inconveniences, sufferings, and misunderstandings that they had endured. This was also the moment when I realized that Zuleana® was for everybody. I gained a special affinity for women who were what I call my, *"Heavy Duty Cuties."* These are women who are 300-500 pounds.

Testimony #3

(The student steps on the scale and screams.)

Student: YES! YES! YES! I did it! I did it!

Me: What happened, babe?

Student: I am 199 pounds!

Me: Okay, and?

Student: Coach. I made it! I made it into the 100's. I have never been in the 100's since I was a child! I will never ever have to see that "2" ever again. I am in the 100s!

(I ring my cowbell and do my happy dance. The students scream and shout and do crazy-cool movements in Zuleana® "drop pounds" celebration style.)

Testimony #4

Student: Coach, I will be able to buy my scale soon!

Me: Baby, why don't you go ahead and buy a scale today? Don't be afraid of the scale, babe.

Student: Oh, no. I'm not afraid. A regular scale doesn't weigh past four hundred and I am almost there! I will finally be able to buy me a scale and weigh myself in my own home.

I am so excited! Just 22 more pounds down and I will be able to buy my own scale, Coach Cee Cee!

I can't even handle moments like this. I just look away, trying to be cool but my heart won't allow it. It swells up once again with hope, faith, love, patience, understanding, and pure joy. I am in awe of these women, of what they are becoming. I am taken aback, a bit bewildered, and completely stunned by the transformations that stand before me. I am undone by my own well doing. Lord, You are so amazingly good to all of us. Thank You, Lord, for Your grace, mercy, wisdom, and of course, Zuleana®.

The Power of Reishi Mushroom Tea
(Ganoderma lucidum)

Reishi is an edible Chinese medicinal fungus (mushroom)…crazy, right? This mushroom tea is a powerful anti-inflammatory. You already know-it's available in my online store.

Here are just a few of reishi's benefits:

- Helps autoimmune disorders and diabetes

- Fights Inflammation, aches, and pains

- Fights cancer/tumors

- Boost Immunity/flu/HIV/AIDS/hepatitis

- Improves liver/liver disease

- Helps heart disease, high blood pressure, high cholesterol

- Alleviates stress and depression

- Improves mental clarity

- Fights against food allergies, asthma, and sinus

- Fights infection (bronchitis, respiratory, urinary tract, skin disorders, etc.)

- Helps digestive problems, ulcers, leaky gut syndrome

- Helps sleep disorders and insomnia

The Power of Mangosteen Tea

Mangosteen is a rare, tropical, purple fruit from Thailand that is incredibly significant to our health. The tea is made from the rind of the mangosteen fruit and has a super- rich, smooth taste. It is best known for its cancer- fighting properties. I can't keep this "so called" secret tea on the shelves. People absolutely adore this Thai treasure.

Mangosteen tea's benefits include:

- Heals skin infections
- Helps intestinal issues
- Anti-cancer
- Blocks bacterial and fungi growth
- Anti-oxidant, anti-bacterial, and anti-tumor
- Provides overall well-being and longevity
- Heals cell damage
- Boosts red blood cells
- Aids anemia
- Provides dilation of blood vessels/fights against strokes, coronary heart disease, and blood pressure

Zuleana® Cheat Sheet

Okay. Not really. But it is quite sneaky in a super-smart kind of way!

1. The yolk of a boiled egg is 55 calories while the egg white is only 15 calories. So, we take the yolk out of the second egg to save us 55 calories, which we then replace with 55 calories of healthy veggies.

2. We add Ceylon cinnamon, turmeric, and Vitamineral Green™ powder (located in my online store) to our matcha powder to add more fat-burning and nutritionally-dense superfood power in the morning.

3. We eat ½ cup of blueberries on top of our oatmeal almost every morning. Blueberries help fight against bad cholesterol, heart disease, diabetes, intestinal upsets, eye disease, and cancer.

4. If we know we are going to eat brown rice (high carb) for dinner, we will skip on eating one of our apples or not eat an apple at all on that day. Or, we might just eat a piece of fruit and a boiled egg for breakfast instead of eating oatmeal (high carb) that day. We keep our carb intake nice and low.

5. We only eat a very small sweet potato (high carb) or a bit of pineapple (high sugar) or water melon (high sugar) once a week or every two weeks.

6. We only eat ½ of a banana when we eat them, which is only about twice a week, if that.

7. We drink and eat lots of organic turmeric powder on our brown rice, cauliflower rice, boiled eggs, salad dressings, tuna, and salmon. Turmeric helps fight fat and inflammation!

8. If we go one day without a bowel movement, we know to increase our fiber intake. We also know that our bowel movements should be about 7 inches long (or more) for maximum detoxification.

9. We squeeze lots of lemon and lime in our water at all times and drink 10 or more glasses of water a day. We try our best to drink ½ of our body weight in ounces on a daily basis.

10. We realize that Zuleana® consists of medicinal herbal teas which are gentle yet potent. Real herbs, and not just (dead) flavors or harsh laxative-concoctions like many of the average teas sold at American grocers.

11. We consume the DE white detox powder for as long as possible, keeping it close at hand. It gets rid of parasites, fungi, bacteria, yeast, and most importantly…**heavy metals!**

12. For anti-cancer and anti-fibroid's sake, we make sure all plastics are BPA-free! BPA stands for bisphenol A and is an industrial chemical used to make certain plastics such as water bottles, food storage containers, and plastic sandwich bags. We do not cook with aluminum foil. We use stainless steel or cast-iron pans. We don't use a lot of lotions, perfumes, powders, bubble bath, and sprays on our bodies. We don't burn candles (chemicals). Instead, we burn essential oils or use essential oil mist to freshen up a room.

13. We do not consume canola oil. It is made from the rape seed plant and is not as healthy for the body as other oils. We rely on olive oil, coconut oil, and fish oils.

14. Grapes mold easily and berries don't like moisture. Take the grapes and berries out of the bags and containers, gently wash, pat dry, place in a single layer on a paper towel in an open container, and place in the refrigerator.

15. Citrus fruits are best kept on the counter. Instead of displaying them in a fruit bowl, simply place the pieces of fruit on the counter a bit apart from one another to resist mold growth.

16. We cook our gluten-free oatmeal on top of the stove. Sometimes we cook a few cups at night, store away, and reheat in the morning. But if we heat up an item in the microwave, we use GLASS bowls not plastic storage containers. **Repeat:** USE GLASS or CERAMIC BOWLS IN THE MICROWAVE.

The Zuleana® Girl Life

- There are days when a Zuleana® girl will simply not eat meat at all.

- A Zuleana® girl does not have to eat until she is stuffed. She can stop eating when she is 80% full.

- When ordering a salad, a Zuleana® girl will request to place her cheese on the side (we are only allowed to eat feta or goat cheese) and then place like five tiny sprinkles on her salad.

- Zuleana® girls know that wheat is dangerous to our health. It is addictive and can be an appetite stimulant. Pasta and bread are big trouble in the Zuleana® way. The gluten that wheat contains can cause numerous health issues.

- Zuleana® girls realize the dangers of consuming soy. Most soy in America is genetically modified. It is hidden in veggie, patties, protein shakes, protein bars, and cooking spray-it's everywhere. Beware, soy can damage your thyroid, your metabolism, and your hormones.

- A Zuleana® girl knows that regular/conventional cow's milk can contain steroids, pesticides, antibiotics, and even bacteria from infected animals. Instead, we drink 30 calories, unsweetened, organic almond milk.

- A Zuleana® girl will have faith, pray to God for healing, and then put in the work to help heal her body with natural medicine and wise food choices.

- A Zuleana® girl is excited about going to the doctor with great expectation to get a copy of her lab results.
- A Zuleana® girl is very familiar with her blood work and lab result numbers such as glucose, A1c, hydroxy D3, blood pressure, iron level, and thyroid level.

The Numbers You Need to Know!

- A1c should be 5.5 and lower

- Blood glucose should be 95 and lower

  (100-125mg/dl is considered pre-diabetic)

- Hemoglobin (Iron level) should be 13.5-17.5

- Cholesterol total should be less than 200

- HDL (good) should be 60-70

- LDL (bad) should be 100 or lower

- Blood pressure should be 120 over 80

- TSH (thyroid test) should be 0.2-5.0

  (under 0.5 is hyperthyroid and over 5.0 is hypothyroid)

- Find out your blood type and remember it

ZULEANA® GIRLS REALIZE THERE IS SO MUCH MORE TO GREAT HEALTH THAN SMOOTHIES AND SHAKES. WE ARE KNOWN FOR DRINKING POWERFUL SPICE ELIXIRS. WE MIX, WHISK, STIR, AND SHAKE. WE CREATE OUR OWN

NATURAL MEDICINE

#Zuleana

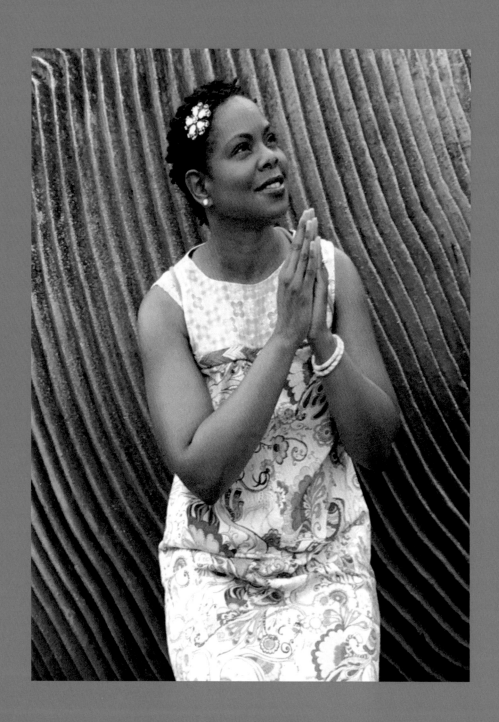

Jehovah Rapha

Humble yourself and pray and He will come and heal. Remember the Lord, Our God is the one who heals. By His stripes we are already healed. That is His promise.

It's good to call Him by one of His particular identities and that is Rapha. RAPHA means to restore, to heal, to make healthful (in Hebrew.) Jehovah Rapha can be translated as "Jehovah Who Heals." He is the Great Physician who heals your physical and emotional needs. Cry out to Jehovah Rapha, have no doubt, and watch His healing power. If you have cried out to Jesus time and time again, get a little more personal and pull on his healing heartstrings. Stand on His healing promises and meditate on His word. Call on Him with all of your attention and with a very (focused faith) on total healing. Lastly, declare that He will perfect your concerns and do a mighty work in you, right now! Keep your faith alive. Never stop believing that He can and He will heal you. By your faith, you are healed!

Live Like an Okinawan

The women of Okinawa, Japan, are the longest living women in the entire world. Here are a few Okinawan secrets that I have incorporated into Zuleana®.

- We eat a sweet potato, purple potato, or Japanese potato at least once a week.
- We eat seaweed by eating miso soup or seaweed salad found at Japanese restaurants here in America. (Note: Ask for more seaweed and little to no tofu.)
- We drink Vitamineral Greens™ powder which contains 6 types of seaweed: dulse, nori, kelp, alaria, bladderwrack and laver.
- We eat lots of turmeric and garlic.
- We drink green tea. We prefer one of the hightest grades of green tea called matcha. We drink ½ teaspoon in 8 ounces of water with a bit of turmeric.
- We eat Shitake mushrooms.

Have an Elephant Mentality

NEVER FORGET TO EAT:

- Cauliflower rice instead of brown rice
- Cauliflower mashed potatoes
- Miso soup
- Brussels sprouts
- Apricots
- 13 cherries
- Bok choy
- Radish
- 3 oz. of grass-fed, organic lamb
- Bragg 24 Herbs & Spices
- Asparagus
- Fennel, rosemary, parsley, thyme, and parsley
- Butternut squash
- Zucchini
- ½ Pear
- Small apple
- 3 slices of avocado

Dangers of Aluminum

Aluminum is a heavy metal. Many times aluminum is found in our deodorant. It can seep through our lymph system and travel straight to the breast causing possible breast cancer and other complications. If you simply take a look at the ingredients of your deodorant, you will see the high aluminum percentages that it contains. This same aluminum is what stains your beautiful white shirts in the armpit area and even stains/darkens your skin under the armpit. This can be very disheartening. Many times boils that grow under your armpits are from the accumulation of aluminum and other chemicals from deodorants. Start using a non-aluminum deodorant. I have a great herbal deodorant in my online store on my website. It is great for men, women, boys, and girls of all ages and yes, it works!

#nomorealuminum

Endometriosis Care

- Eliminate dairy foods

- Eliminate whey

- Eliminate casein

- Eliminate cow's milk

- Eliminate milk protein (usually found in protein shakes)

- Eliminate soy

- Avoid alcohol

- Eat organic foods

- Eat hormone-free meats

- Take a fish oil pill

- Drink red raspberry leaf tea twice daily

- Get more B6, selenium, and *magnesium

- Take *vitex 800-1,000 mg (chaste tree capsule)

Note: Do not take chaste tree if you are on birth control pills or other hormonal drugs. Try your best not to take a huge amount of contraceptive pills and pain-killers as this can damage the balance in your digestive system.

*These items are located in my online store.

Missing Gallbladder Care

The gallbladder secretes lots of bile into your intestines after a fatty meal. Bile is a way for your body to excrete toxins and waste. A healthy gallbladder helps your body excrete cholesterol, fats, and fat soluble toxins. People without a gallbladder are more prone to have liver and digestive problems. Stones can still form within the ducts of the liver. You could also develop a fatty liver.

If you eat a fatty meal, the fat will not digest well because there is not enough bile. This means you may experience bloating, nausea, diarrhea, and indigestion. You may not digest fats well such as essential fatty acids (EFAs) and fat soluble vitamins such as vitamins A, D, E and K. So will most likely need some supplements. ***Digestive enzyme therapy is highly recommended for anyone who does not have a gallbladder***. *I have helped so many women, who have missing gallbladders acquire major restoration with my Zuleana® better health consultation.*

So let's get further understanding. If you are having problems with your gallbladder, it's because you have an unhealthy liver. This means your liver may be producing poor quality bile. This kind of bile is likely to form sludge and stones. Here is a list of helpful suggestions.

- **DAIRY IS A NO-NO!** Milk, cheese, ice cream, and yogurt worsen all cases of gallbladder disease and liver disease. These foods are very difficult to digest.

- **GRAINS ARE A NO-NO!** Gluten intolerance is common among those with missing gallbladders. By keeping your grains low, this will lower your risk of developing fatty liver.

- **DRINK *MILK THISTLE, DANDELION ROOT TEA (found in *Ojibwa tea) and *ARTICHOKE LEAF TEA.**

- Take a good quality **OX BILE SUPPLEMENT with each meal.** This will help with indigestion, bloating, diarrhea, and other symptoms.

- Take a **DIGESTIVE ENZYME.** It helps reduce indigestion, intestinal bacteria growth, and candida.

- Take *Vitamin D3 (5000IU)** with a bit of good fat such as avocado or olive oil. It is much harder for the D3 capsules to absorb in those who have missing gallbladders so on some days, you may want to take two Vitamin D3 capsules.

* These items can be found in my online store.

Secret #6:
The Blessing of Nutritional Yeast

This is not the kind of yeast that causes candida or cause any problems with people who have yeast overgrowth, so never fear. This is a wonderful seasoning made of sugar cane and beet molasses that can be used on soups and salads. This yeast is packed with 17 vitamins and 14 minerals. It is truly one of the most powerful superfoods I have come across in my medicine hunting. It is protein-rich, low in fat, and easily digested. It has all nine essential amino acids and gives your food a bit of a cheesy/meat-like taste. I like the Bragg brand the best as they fortified it with vitamin B12. This makes it great for vegetarians who need more vitamin B12. Nutritional yeast also provides beta-glucan so it will also help with lowering bad cholesterol. It builds the immune system and it is anti-viral and anti-bacterial. It also contains selenium, which helps fight cancer.

Secret #7:
Blackstrap Molasses

- Blackstrap molasses is great for increasing your iron level, especially needed for blood loss and heavy menstruations.

- It contains huge amounts of calcium.

- It includes manganese.

- It includes copper.

- It contains magnesium, selenium, and B6.

Molasses Milk Recipe

8 oz. of warm almond milk
1 teaspoon of black strap molasses
½ teaspoon of Ceylon cinnamon
1 teaspoon of organic ginger powder
1 tablespoon of raw honey
Several ice cubes

Put all the ingredients into a blender and mix until completely combined.

Note: You can warm the milk and mixture on the stove (low heat) if you prefer the drink warm. You can also add molasses (1 tablespoon) to a cup of warm water, oatmeal, or a hemp protein shake. Be sure to buy *organic, unsulphured molasses.*

Secret #8:

Zuleana® Vinaigrette Salad Dressing

Zuleana® DIY Citrus Salad Dressing

1 tablespoon Bragg Apple Cider Vinegar
2 tablespoons extra virgin olive oil
1 tablespoon fresh herbs
½ -1 teaspoon Bragg Organic 24 Herbs & Spices
1 organic lime
1 organic tangerine
Pinch of Himalayan salt and black pepper

Put all the ingredients, with salt and pepper to taste, into a blender bottle (shaker with whisk ball) and shake thoroughly, then pour over your salad. **You can switch out the citrus for berries if you want a berry-based dressing.**

Note that we don't fry or stir-fry with olive oil, we only use EVO on top of salads. We always stir-fry with 100% MCT extra virgin coconut oil. Coconut oil can handle the highest of cooking heat and is incredibly healthy for the brain (Alzheimer's). The liver processes coconut oil easily, so it is converted to energy instead of fat.

More About Coconut Oil

Coconut oil has so many mind-blowing benefits. Don't ever let anyone talk you out of consuming your coconut oil. The ketones in coconut oil creates a source of energy to help repair brain function.

- Helps with UTI, kidney Infections, and the liver
- Fights helicobacter pylori (stomach issue/cancer)
- Enhances immune system
- Reduces inflammation, arthritis, osteoporosis
- Prevents heart disease and high blood pressure
- Helps Alzheimer's patients
- Improves brain function and memory
- Improves energy and endurance
- Improves ulcerative colitis
- Improves digestion and stomach ulcers
- Helps with dandruff and itchy skin
- Helps weight loss, decrease appetite, and burn belly fat
- Helps balance hormones (great for menopause)

Zuleana®

Makes Your Skin Beautiful

Here is a list of elements in our eating lifestyle and some activities that make the skin gorgeous.

- Avocados
- Blueberries, blackberries, raspberries, strawberries
- Pumpkin and sunflower seeds
- Wild caught salmon
- Raw almonds
- Artichoke leaf tea
- Ojibwa tea and /or liver cleanse tea
- Lemon, limes, and grapefruit
- Pomegranate seeds
- Dark chocolate
- Spinach
- Extra virgin olive oil
- Coconut oil (Consume it and rub into the skin.)
- Carrots
- Apples
- Hemp protein
- Get 7 hours of sleep nightly and exercise 5-6 days a week

Zuleana®
Takes Care of Your Brain

Here are several elements in our lifestyle that will help with memory, brain fog, mental performance, and Alzheimer's disease.

- Blueberries
- Wild caught salmon and sardines
- Almonds and seeds
- Avocados
- Beets and celery
- Coconut oil
- Dark chocolate
- Miso soup
- Broccoli and cauliflower
- Bone broth
- Herbs such as rosemary, oregano, sage, and peppermint
- Turmeric and ashwagandha
- Ginkgo biloba and ginseng
- Spinach, kale, swiss chard, and romaine lettuce
- Egg yolk and grapefruit (provides choline)
- Matcha green tea (provides L-theanine)

Cancer Care

It is my prayer that every human being realizes the power of **apoptosis**-the process by which cells destroy themselves! **#cellsuicide**

- **Sour Sop leaves**
- **Ojibwa tea**
- **Curcumin/Turmeric (powder and capsules)**
- **Matcha green tea**
- **Astragalus (tea or capsules)**
- **Cat's Claw**
- **Milk Thistle**
- **Pau D'Arco**
- **Sweet Wormwood (Chinese herb)**
- **Supplements such as selenium, vitamin D3, and resveratrol**
- **Grape seed extract**
- **Chlorella and wheatgrass**

Note: I have an anti-cancer, 6-piece care kit in my online store. I also encourage you to do your own research. Some of the above elements may conflict with some drugs. Please check with your medical doctor before use.

A Reflection: The Will

I can't stand when someone gives another a negative report saying, "You have so many weeks or months to live." Are you serious? Who made that person the father of time?

I serve a living God who happens to be amazing with time. Not only is He is a master creator, He is known for being an incredible redeemer of all things. He is also known for miraculously returning valuables that have been stolen like joy, vitality, and life itself.

I have noticed one thing in my 23 years of helping the so-called "forgotten ones." You don't even have to feel like you can make it, just simply have *the will* to live. My God loves a willing vessel and He tends to use those kinds of vessels quickly. He will turn it around for your good. Your (second-chance) life will exceed your every expectation and the body, which has been wonderfully and fearfully made, will do what it has always been created to do—heal itself!

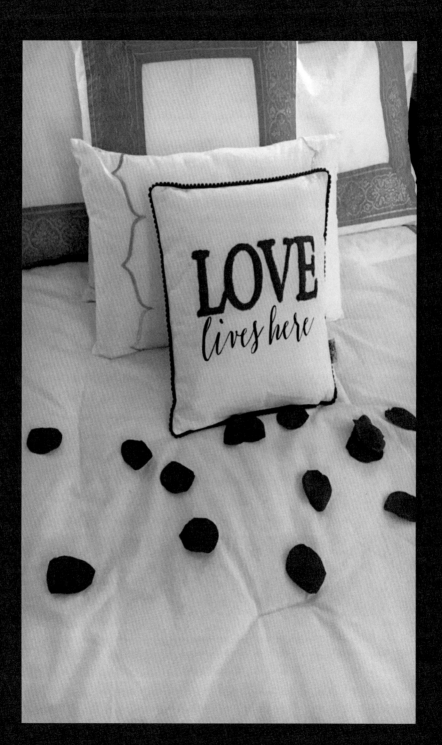

The Marriage Bed

Here are few elements that will support hormonal balance and female libido.

- Maca

- Ashwaganda

- Vitex

- Damiana

- Yohimbe

- Dark chocolate

- Eat fish from the STASH-T list

Note: In the case of infertility, <u>maca is awesome for both males and females.</u> The ladies might also try taking royal jelly capsules, alleviate coffee, red meat, and processed foods. Be sure to drink a bit of ginkgo biloba/green tea (It's called Think Sharp tea from my website.) Ginkgo biloba helps balance estrogen and progesterone. You should also make sure your iron level is high. Low iron may dim your libido.

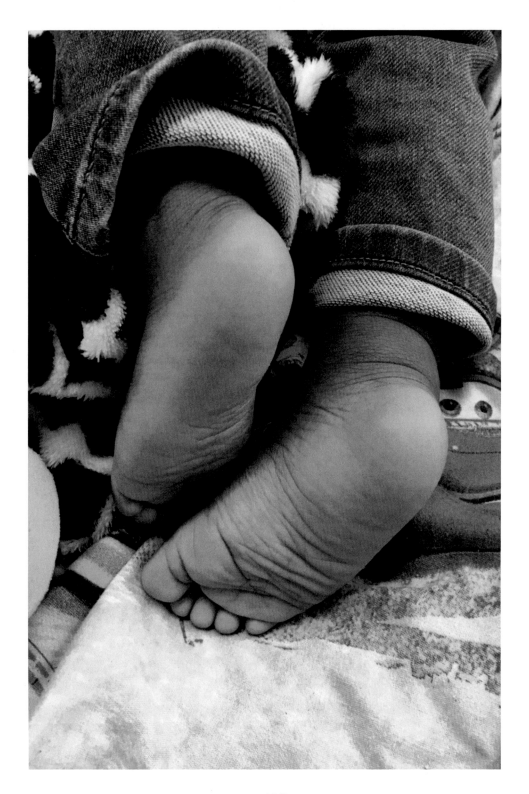

Zuleana Poem #3: Little One

You, little one, will not have to go through

What I have been through

Your world will be cleaner

Brighter

Your grass will be much greener than mine

I am starting anew

Tender mercy was waiting for me

And I grabbed hold of it

What I eat, you will eat

And you will grow big and strong and tall

like a palm tree

You will bend but you will not break

I have found a new way

and everything is going to be okay

Now that I know

The *"way"*

Surround Yourself with Thinkers

Take time out to **BE INSPIRED!** Life is nothing without inspiration, so here is a list of people who inspire me.

- Jesus Christ
- Harriet Tubman
- Maya Angelou
- Benjamin Franklin
- Helen Keller
- Anne Sullivan
- Derek Prince
- Michelle Obama
- Nelson Mandela
- Desmond Tutu
- Kate Spade
- Martha Stewart
- Ellen Degeneres
- Daymond John
- Alvin Ailey
- Martha Graham
- Albert Einstein
- Vincent Van Gogh
- Georgia O'Keefe
- Lori Greiner

- Misty Copeland
- Frederick Douglass
- Rev. Dr. Martin Luther King, Jr.
- Nicholas Sparks
- Madame C.J. Walker
- Debbie Allen
- Lilly Singh
- Alicia Keys
- Malala Yousafzay
- Tina Turner
- Kendra Scott
- George C. Wolfe
- Oprah Winfrey
- Boaz
- Ruth
- Esther
- Audrey Hepburn
- Thomas Edison
- Anne Frank

- Barbara Walters
- Dallas Shaw
- Anne Fontaine
- Stevie Wonder
- Langston Hughes
- John W. Nordstrom
- Bruce Nordstrom
- Edgar Degas
- Debbie Allen
- Barbra Streisand
- Philip Freelon
- Paul R. Williams
- Noah Webster
- Judy Blume
- Mary Baxter
- Henrietta Lacks
- Rosa Parks
- Phillis Wheatley
- Thurgood Marshall
- Oliver L. Brown
- Ruby Bridges
- Zora Neale Hurston
- Tracey Reese
- Michael Jackson
- Katherine Johnson
- Gregory Hines
- Chimamanda Ngozi Adichie
- Lucille Ball
- Carol Burnett
- Amalia Eriksson
- Chris Anderson
- Steven Covey
- Bruce McPherson
- Hayne Hipp
- Cherington Shucker
- Nick Vujicic
- Ann Fonta
- Truett Cathy
- Hippocrates
- Wilbert Floyd
- My mom, Vivian Patterson

Zuleana® on the Go

I know many of you are out saving the world and making big things happen. So I hooked you up with a handy-dandy list.

Zuleana® Approved Restaurants

- **Panera Bread**
- **Zoe's Kitchen**
- **Jason's Deli**
- **Grabbagreen**
- **B. good**
- **Happy + Hale**
- **First Watch**
- **Chopt**

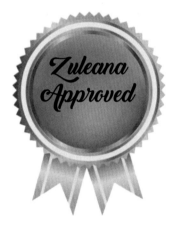

- **Tropical Smoothie Café (Ask for the Detox Island Green™ smoothie.)**
- **Ruby Tuesday (salad bar or kale salad)**
- **Chipotle (Ask for brown rice and no shell)**
- **Outback Steakhouse and Longhorn- salmon/broccoli**
- **Apple Bee's–lemon chicken dish w/ side of spinach**
- **Red Robin–salmon with broccoli (bottomless)**
- **Earth Fare–hot bar/salad bar/juice bar**
- **Whole Foods–hot bar/salad bar**
- **Mellow Mushroom-build our own salad**

Zuleana® While at Hotels

Almost every hotel has the following accommodations, so use them.

- Pool

- Sauna

- Gym Equipment

- Oatmeal in the morning

- Apples in the lobby

- Water with lemon/lime in the lobby

- Coffee maker for heating water

- A refrigerator for your bottled water and fruit

Zuleana® Poem #4: With My Tears

Don't talk behind my back,

talk to my back because I am leaving the past

behind. I have chosen to follow Him!

You have the spirit of Peninnah.

You doubt me worse than Thomas

and you have already denied me three times.

I will not be your pillar of salt!

I see my future — the open door.

Patience and Kindness will be my welcome mat

Hope and Joy will be waiting for me on the inside.

We will sit at the table and laugh

until I cry

and wipe His feet with my tears.

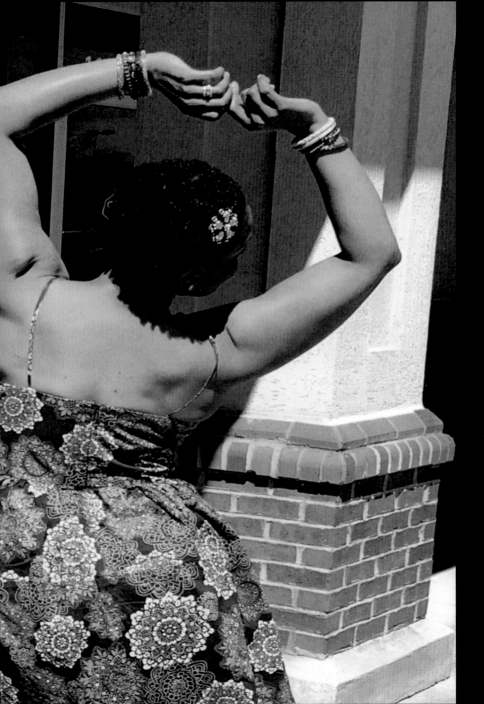

Too Blessed to be Stressed

Stress is a killer and is one of the key culprits of cancer and countless other discomforts and diseases. Here are some ideas to try for de-stressing.

- Grow your own garden.

- Take a little walk every hour while at work

- Go get massages and practice deep breathing.

- Resolve issues early, don't go to bed in anger.

- Close your eyes and visualize yourself whole and at peace.

- Draw, color, or paint even if you don't know how!

- Learn to just say "no" and "enough is enough."

- Eat de-stressing foods that support adrenal gland function as brown rice, algae, cabbage, almonds, berries, celery, sunflower seeds, cucumbers, asparagus, garlic, and avocados.

- Stop eating foods that cause stress such as alcohol, sweets, salty foods, cow's milk, red meat, refined and processed foods, margarine, spicy foods, and caffeine found in coffee and sodas.

- **FORGIVE EVERYONE!** Unforgiveness, bitterness, and resentment can lodge in the body and cause major sickness and disease. In Matthew 18:21-35 it tells us that if we don't forgive people, we get turned over to the torturers. Whew, the *Word of God is quick, powerful, and sharp!*

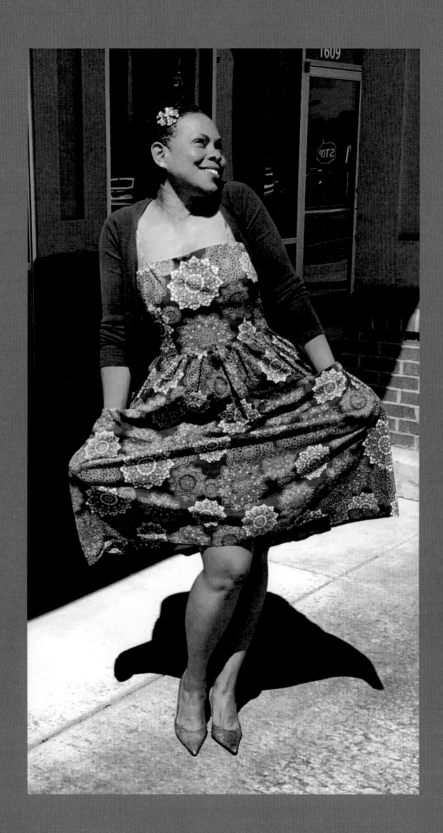

Final Dangers

1. **MSG** (monosodium glutamate) is an excitotoxin that over excites the cells to the point of damage, even brain damage. MSG also puffs up the body. MSG can cause headaches, migraines, and stomach upset. **Google: MSG induced mice**

2. **Lectins** are a type of protein that can bind to cell membranes. They can causes bloating, gas, indigestion, and major damage to the gastrointestinal tract. The highest quantities of lectins are found in **WHEAT** and **BEANS**.

3. **Isoflavones** are found in **SOY**. This **anti**-nutrient can cause harmful hormonal changes and digestive issues. Look for hidden soy in protein shakes, protein bars, veggie burgers, and cooking oils in spray cans.

4. **GMO** (genetically modifies organism) is the result of when the DNA of one species is artificially forced into the genes of an unrelated plant or animal. **In Zuleana®, due to harmful GMOs, we do not eat corn, cow's milk, or any artificial sweetners.**

5. **Phthalate** are found in plastics, perfume, cosmetics, shampoo, lotion and nail polish. They can be damaging to the lungs, liver, kidney, and reproductive system. Ladies with PCOS and endometriosis must be very leery of phthalates.

The *power*

is in the

leaves!

The leaves of the trees were for the **healing** of the nations.

Rev. 22:2

Zuleana® Poem #5: Kissed By The Sun

To my sisters who have been

kissed by the sun.

You must remember to take time out for yourself.

You are the mothers of the earth,

You have taken care of your children and

other people's children.

You are so very strong yet,

sometimes feel weak.

Where has your smile gone to my dear?

We are so blessed and we have come so far.

Let us remember our history.

It runs so wide and so deep

who can even comprehend it?

We use to wade in the water together, my sister,

running from this hound and that hound.

Now we can swim together freely

from Havasu Falls, Macarella Beach, to the

Nile River in Africa.

See, they captured us in West Africa.

West Africans are known to be some of the best

swimmers, divers, and fisherman.

We brought these skills with us as slaves.

We use to bend and pick the cotton

making sure we did not look master in the eye

but keep our heads bent low and backs

deeply, curved over the cotton fields.

Stand up straight my sister, smell the fresh air and turn

your face to the sun.

Say hello to your day, my love.

Do not be afraid of the sun for the sun is

so in love with you!

Its energy travels ninety-three million miles just to touch

your beautiful skin, my love.

Did you not know?

See, there is a time to use great discretion,

when you must be wise as a serpent

and innocent as a dove.

Then there are times when you must speak out.

Speak out loud and clear for what you believe in.

Your voice carries, my sister.

Your voice carries like

a djembe drum or the talking drum carrying signals to the next village that carried it to the next village and the next.

Messages that were transmitted at the speed of 100 miles an hour, secret rhythmic code that travelled faster than the Europeans who were trying to capture them. Yes! We made drums talk, chile!

We are some of the greatest communicators in all of the universe.

Everything about us speaks my love.

Our backs talk, our legs sing, and the sway of our hips will sho' nuff tell you stories that will make you lean in, listen, and learn.

You, my sister, are more powerful than you know!

Your hair does a daily dance with its twists and turns, coils and curls.

It bounces and snaps and sticks up and out as if curious about the world.

Your ends are not split but strong, standing straight up surveying the situation searching for your next move.

Yes, our hair springs up and out

singing songs of love and happiness and you

must continue to encourage yourself.

But today,

let me encourage you my love, my dear.

Sister, let me tell you how you beautiful you are.

The gap in your teeth is perfect.

The sway in your back is perfect.

The flatness of the arch in your foot is…

YES! Perfect!

The black of your eye is gorgeous like a beautiful

sunflower shooting up above all the other flowers.

The lily of the valley wishes she could be as strong and

beautiful as you, baby!

You are sun-kissed by design

Yes, you have been kissed by the sun

You came out of the womb with kisses all over you

Kissed by the Son.

You are lovely indeed, something worth waiting for.

For you I would wait a thousand years hoping that a

thousand years would become one day

just to be with you.

You, my sister, are like rubies... so very rare.

Let diamonds be your best friend because you are a

ruby, my love. Did they not tell you?

You are the super to my natural.

The raw to my honey

the honey to my bee

The be to my come

and you are becoming

who you really want to be!

Every day is a chance to simply

become.

There is a time to be

and then there is a time to...

become

whatever it is that you were born to be

because you have a purpose in this world.

You have a place.

Be careful who fills your space

and who is that in your ear, my sister?

Because faith comes by hearing.

Don't you know your time is valuable?

Manage it well my love, manage it well.

Your world is being created every minute

every moment so...

dust off your vision

polish your dreams

keep shaping who you are because

You are special,

beautifully different

and very unique.

Has anyone not told you?

Shame on all of them because

everything about you is exquisite

simply because you, my dear sister,

have been

kissed by the sun.

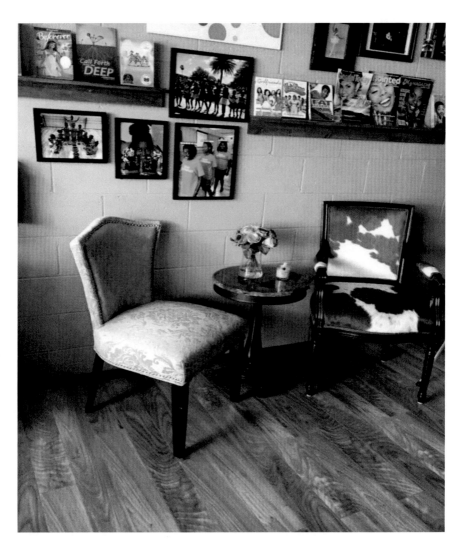

This was my former creativity studio, located in Greenville, SC, where many health consultations took place. Many needs were met and lives were changed.

#createbetterhealth

#hardwoodfloorbysweethubby
#thecarpenterswife

My Passion For
NATURAL MEDICINE

I have had the pleasure of helping women with rare and sometimes debilitating diseases such as:

- Takayasu arteritis–(2.6 cases per million population) is a chronic inflammation of the large blood vessels that distribute blood from the heart, including the aorta and its main branches

- Ankylosing Spondylitis–(200,000 cases per year) is an inflammatory arthritis affecting the spine and large joints

- Von Willebrand disease –(200,000 cases a year) – is a bleeding disorder

I absolutely have a passion for KILLING DISEASE, NATURALLY! Many of the ladies and their husbands find that after just a few weeks of eating the Zuleana® way, their cholesterol, diabetes, and blood pressure become normal. Many have testified that they no longer find the need to take insomnia, anxiety, or headache medicines. Some share with me that they no longer have to take hormone therapy because the clean eating style and supplements of Zuleana® balance their hormones naturally. This kind of feedback from my customers makes me very happy.

Cee Cee Michaela

THE MEDICINE HUNTER

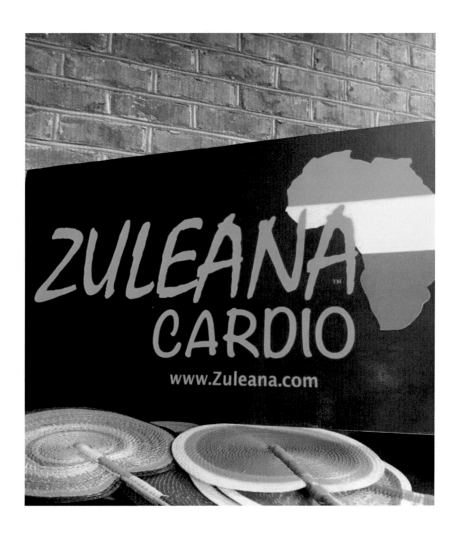

I usually present Zuleana® Cardio when I am invited to speak at universities and women's conferences as well as my own Zuleana® getaways and gatherings. Each lady starts my warm up with a beautiful fan from Nigeria. It is truly an exercise celebration.

#Zuleanafans

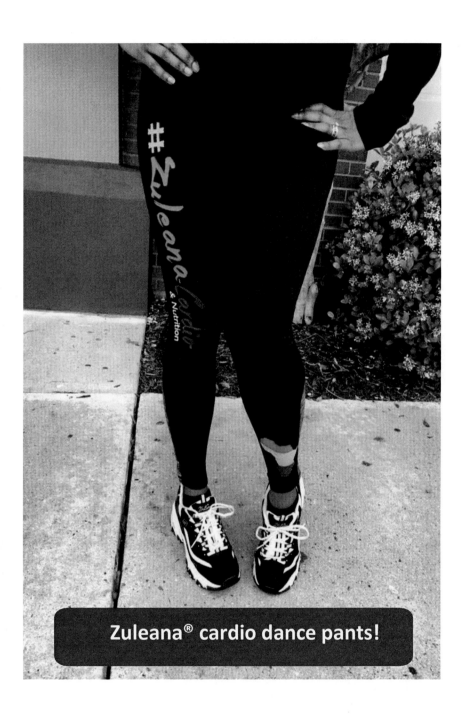

Zuleana® cardio dance pants!

About The Author

Cee Cee Michaela has been living a healthy lifestyle for more than twenty-three years and is known as the *"Harriet Tubman of Health" and "The Weight Loss Coach."* She has traveled and inspired people around the world with her healthy eating seminars. Now, she has perfected her very own weight loss system, African cardio dance technique and cutting-edge healthy eating lifestyle, which all fall under her exciting brand called *Zuleana®*. She is a graduate of the Boston Conservatory of Music. As a successful actress, Cee Cee has graced the stages of Broadway, performing alongside the late Gregory Hines, in Jelly's Last Jam, directed by two-time, Tony Award-winning director George C. Wolfe. She has starred in several movies and numerous television shows such as "All My Children," "The Fresh Prince of Bel Air," and "The Steve Harvey Show." She is probably best known for her character of the zany cop, Yvonne, on the hit TV comedy, "Girlfriends." As a song writer, she has composed over fifty songs, and owns almost 100% of her masters. Many of the songs have scored very popular TV shows and films. Her song: My Name is Harriet, in honor of the life and history of Harriet Tubman, has received almost one million views on You Tube (search: The Harriet Tubman Song.)

Cee Cee is a sought–after speaker as an abstinence-until marriage-advocate as well as a healthy living enthusiast and natural remedies educator. She is an avid reader and a prodigious researcher. If she is not writing books, she is reading them. As an author, this is her fourth book. Her children's book entitled *The Adventures of Zoe*

Greene is an adorable book about a little African American girl who lives a very adventurous life and spreads the message of healthy eating, exercise, and of course anything that is the color, green! Cee Cee is the founder of ***Project Zoe Greene***, a program for young girls, advocating self-esteem, natural beauty, and healthy living while discovering the wonders of nature and the beauty that surrounds them. Cee Cee has dedicated her life to educating as many people as possible about the power of whole foods, nutrients, vitamins, and minerals, which will enable them to live a vibrant, clean, lean, and disease-free life forever!

She resides with her husband, Wilbert, in lovely Raleigh, NC. Cee Cee's hobbies include collecting books for her private library, enjoying historical river cruises, walking along nature trails, discovering cool things off the beaten path with her hubby, and having matcha green tea parties.

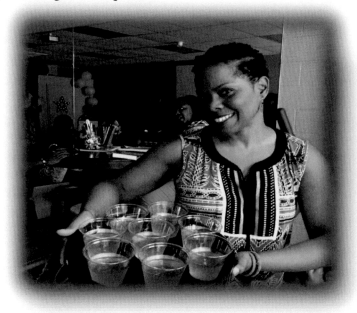

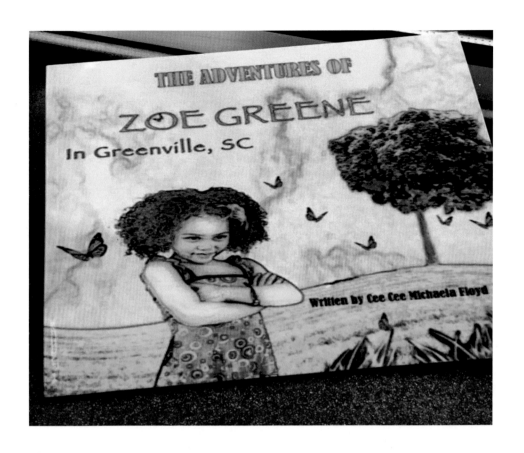

#letsstayconnected

To order a copy of *The Adventures of Zoe Greene*, book Cee Cee for a *speaking engagement*, receive her one-on-one *Zuleana® Better Health and Anti-Disease Consultation*, or find out about the next *Zuleana® Getaway/Conference*, visit her website:

www.IamCeeCee.com
www.Zuleana.com

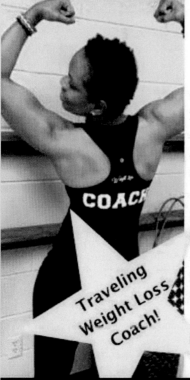

My Personal Style

I love ladylike dresses with touches of vintage and boho accessories. My bracelets were collected from various boutiques across the U.S. Each purchase of a bracelet ensures that girls in Nepal receive support. These bracelets are handmade by the women in Nepal and my purchase helps to rebuild their lives and fight against sex trafficking. **#supportgirls**

My skirt was handmade in Rwanda and purchased at One World Market on 9th street in Durham, NC. It was made by a woman of the Umucyo Sewing Cooperative in Kigali. She used a foot pedal sewing machine. With my purchase, it helped to provide for her family and send her children to school. **#fairtrade**

My headband is practically vintage and is a must for my wild, curly hair. After receiving numerous compliments on my beloved piece, I woke up one morning to a pleasant surprise–several stone headbands handmade by my sweet husband, Wilbert. He is a carpenter, craftsman, and fixer of all broken things around the house. I have decided to sell the headbands on my website in which 50% of the proceeds will go to **PROJECT ZOE GREENE.**

#lovegives   #blesshishands   #craftsmanswife

#happywife   #Zuleanawife   #Zuleanahusband

#Zuleanafamily   #Zuleanaway   #Zuleanalife   #Zuleana

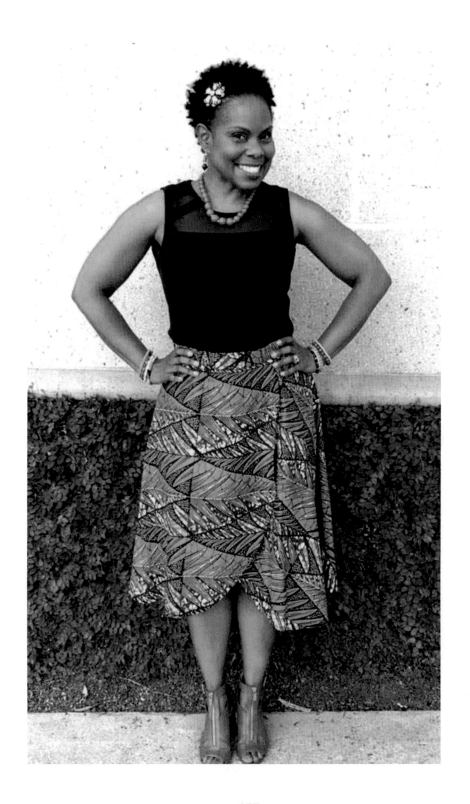

"Sometimes I feel like giving up,

then I think about Harriet Tubman."

–Cee Cee Michaela

They call me the ***"Harriet Tubman of Health."*** I do not take this lightly because she was a very courageous and honorable revolutionary woman, an indelible staple in human history. A devout Christian, she ushered many slaves to freedom through the Underground Railroad over a period of several years.

During the Civil War, she served as a scout, a spy, and a nurse. She mixed herbs and healed many soldiers who were stricken with dysentery. She led raids and rescued 750 slaves. She helped Susan B. Anthony fight for voting rights and was a prolific speaker. Harriet Tubman opened a care facility for elderly African Americans. Upon her death, it was reported that her last words were, "I go to prepare a place for you."

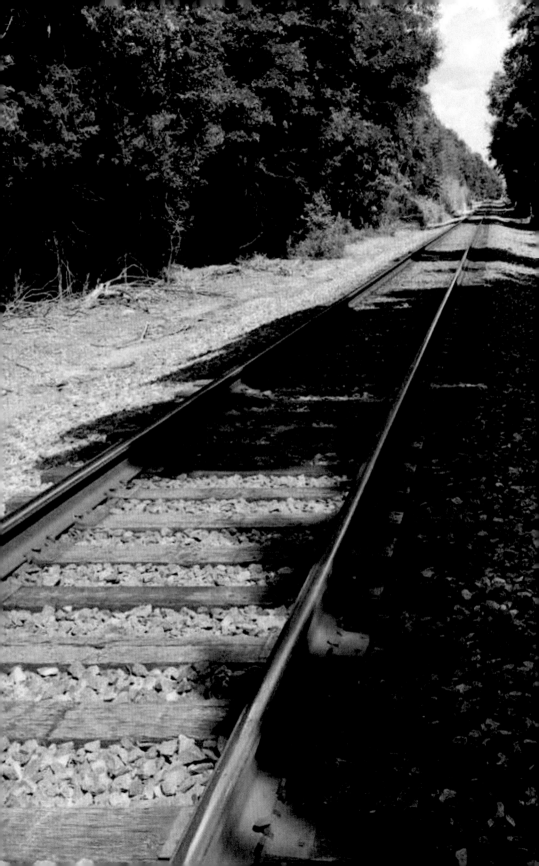

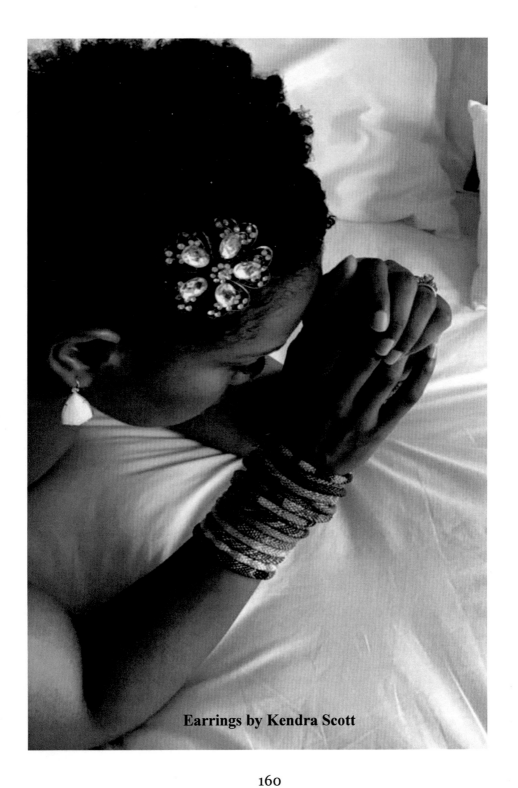

Earrings by Kendra Scott

A Prayer

I think it is no coincidence that you picked up this book. So, if it's okay with you, I'd like to pray for you. I actually end every Zuleana® nutrition/cardio class and conference with a prayer circle. I have found that prayer brings about great hope and miraculous change.

Lord, we call upon you today simply saying thank you! Thank you for waking us up and creating this day for us. Thank you for the sun that shines, the birds that sing, and the air that we breathe. Thank you, Lord, that we are able to see, hear, and feel your presence. You are amazingly loving to all of us. Lord, I ask that you bless the hands that hold this book. Lead and guide them into their purpose. Give them peace and uncommon favor. Perfect everything that concerns them. Send them friends that do not just merely tolerate them but actually celebrate them. Lord, keep us all safe. Shield us from our enemies, hide us under the shadow of your wings and continue to be a fence of protection all around us. Give us your grace and wisdom, Lord. Help us to run this race and to finish strong. I touch and agree with you right now that there be no sickness in your body. All cancers, tumors, cysts, polyps, growths, pain, issues of blood, muscles, tendons, lymph, vessels, arteries, capillaries, tissues, marrow, bones, heart, eyes, ears, nose, throat, intestines, brain, nerves, emotions, all cells, every organ, and all of your bodily systems be completely healed and be made whole, right now! By **His** stripes you are already healed! In *Jesus'* name, we pray. Amen.

A Final Word

Almost all of the medicinal leaves, roots, barks, and seeds can be found in my online store on my website. Many of them are amazing proprietary blends in the form of gentle, yet highly effective, easy-to-drink tea bags and supplements. We are a family-owned business who have consumed and adored these products for years! Our passion is to see other families feeling vibrant, living healthy, celebrating abundance, and experiencing joy because this is how it should be! ;)

XOXO,

CeeCee Michaela

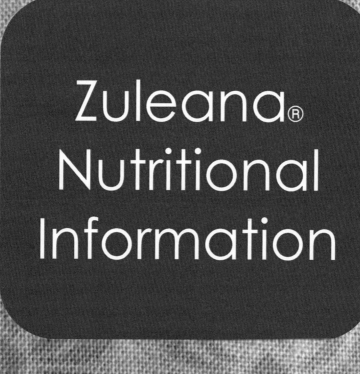

Zuleana® Nutritional Information

The Leaves of Zuleana®

Matcha green tea leaves, Artichoke leaves, Guava leaves, Spinach leaves, Kale leaves, Swiss chard leaves, Collard green leaves Turnip green leaves, Mustard green leaves, Bok choy leaves, Parsley leaves, Basil leaves, Peppermint leaves, Spearmint leaves, Rosemary leaves, Thyme leaves, Cilantro leaves, Fennel leaves, Oolong leaves, Dandelion leaves, Lemongrass leaves, Ginkgo biloba leaves

The Roots of Zuleana®

Turmeric root, Ginger root, Ginseng root, Licorice root, Dandelion root, Turkey Rhubarb root, Maca root, White Peony root Beet root, Chinese Angelica root, Ashwagandha root, Fo-ti root, Astragulus root Lysimachia root, Kutzu root, Isatis root,Tokyo Violet root Duckweed root

The Flowers of Zuleana®

Hibiscus, Chamomille, Jasmine, Red Clover flower Japanese honeysuckle flower, Sophora flower (Liver cleanse tea), Chrysanthemum (Liver cleanse tea)

The Mushrooms of Zuleana®

Reishi (Reishi mushroom tea), Kombucha Shitake

The Barks of Zuleana®

Ceylon cinnamon, Slippery elm bark

The Exotic Medicinal Fruits of Zuleana®

Mangosteen (peel), Acai fruit (inside of the Artichoke leaf tea), Jujube fruit (inside of the Liver cleanse tea), Schisandra fruit

The Stems of Zuleana®

Solomon's Seal, Szechwan Lovage (Menopause tea) Rehmannia (Menopause tea)

The Seeds of Zuleana®

Propolis seed, Fennel seed, Hemp seed, Celosias seed, (Liver cleanse tea)

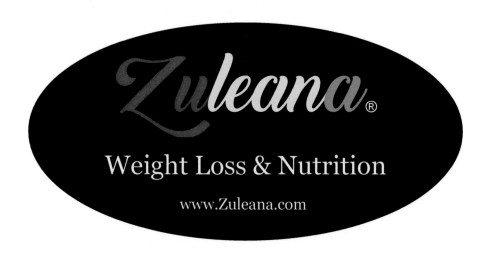

The power of plant-based medicine

"My people are destroyed for lack of knowledge." Hosea 4:6

Let's Socialize!

 Zuleana Lifestyle

 Zuleana and Zoe Life
Cee Cee Michaela

 Cee Cee Michaela

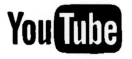 **Zuleana Life TV**

Quantity discounts are available on bulk purchases of this book for educational, gift purchases or as premiums. For information, please e-mail: ceecee@zuleana.com

94621117R00093

Made in the USA
Lexington, KY
01 August 2018